Manifesting Medicine

Artefacts: Studies in the History of Science and Technology

In growing numbers, historians are using technological artefacts in the study and interpretation of the recent past. Their work is still largely pioneering, as they investigate approaches and modes of presentation. But the consequences are already richly rewarding. To encourage this enterprise, three of the world's great repositories of the material heritage of science and technology: the Deutsches Museum, the Science Museum and the Smithsonian Institution, are collaborating on this book series. Each volume treats a particular subject area, using objects to explore a wide range of issues related to science, technology and medicine and their place in society.

Edited by   Robert Bud, Science Museum, London
                 Bernard Finn, Smithsonian Institution, Washington DC
                 Helmuth Trischler, Deutsches Museum, Munich

Volume 1   Manifesting Medicine

                 Principal Editor Robert Bud

Volume 2   Exposing Electronics

                 Principal Editor Bernard Finn

Volume 3   Tackling Transport

                 Principal Editors Helmuth Trischler and Stefan Zeilinger

Volume 4   Presenting Pictures

                 Principal Editor Bernard Finn

Further volumes in preparation, on the themes of:

Military technology
Space

Manifesting Medicine

Edited by

Robert Bud
Science Museum, London

Associate Editors

Bernard Finn
Smithsonian Institution, Washington DC

Helmuth Trischler
Deutsches Museum, Munich

First published 1999 by licence from OPA (Overseas Publishers Association) NV under the Harwood Academic Publishers imprint, part of The Gordon and Breach Publishing Group.

This edition published 2004 by NMSI Trading Ltd, Science Museum, Exhibition Road, London SW7 2DD.

Printed in England by the Cromwell Press.

ISBN 1 900747 56 1
ISSN 1029-3353

Website: http://www.nmsi.ac.uk

Front cover: The Transparent Woman, German Hygiene Museum

Contents

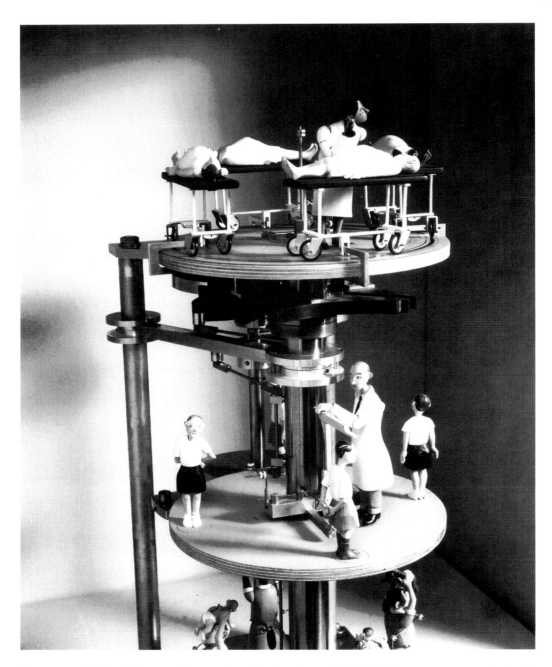

Automaton by Paul Spooner, in carved and painted wood, 1994. The automaton on display in the Science Museum is designed to show that, in the 20th century, medicine has become concerned with the health of whole groups as well as sick individuals. On each level the patients rotate past the medical staff who "automatically" examine them. Science Museum inv. no. 1994–160.

Illustrations

Colour section

Histories, exhibitions, collections

Series Preface

In the long history of the efforts made by science museums to promote the importance of their collections, the past decade has been among the most exciting. Whereas the competition from non-object based science centres has become ever stronger, interest in using objects to communicate insight into the history of our technological and scientific heritage has gained new strength. For millions of visitors, artefacts provide a uniquely attractive and direct link to the past.

Museums also have a research mission. They are a vital force in the community of scholars, especially in the history of technology, and here, too, they have come to be better appreciated. Many outside their walls have come to share the belief that artefacts have played a role which is both inadequately understood and indispensable for a better understanding of historical and cultural change.

Initially, perhaps, it was the insight into technical detail provided by close inspection of the real thing that was generally of greatest scholarly importance. More recently, however, studies of experiments and technology have widened the view to the complex role of artefacts within their larger geographical, economic, social and political setting. Rather than being treated in isolation, technological objects and instruments are coming to be used as material expressions of human culture that shape, mediate and reflect the interactions amongst science, technology and society. Latter-day onlookers are therefore helped to see not just machines, but also imaginative worlds of the past.

Building on rapidly maturing scholarly interest, three of the world's great repositories of material heritage (the Deutsches Museum in Munich, the National Museum of American History in Washington and the Science Museum in London) are cooperating to support this new series of publications. Volumes will explore innovative approaches to the object-oriented historiography of science and technology. The series will seek to go beyond a strict technical description of artefacts on the one hand, and an overly broad social history on the other.

Collections reflect local, regional and national traditions and express their cultures and history. This character confers certain constraints, but also advantages. Museums are sensitive to, and reflect, the specific local meanings of objects, but they have the asset, too, of curators whose detailed knowledge of the collections is couched within a wider historical perspective.

Building on these dual strengths, the series is intended to initiate an international discussion which both emphasizes local material cultures, and also draws upon recent research in the overall history of science and technology. The authors will therefore include curators, but the series will attract into the discussion other scholars from a much wider orbit. Many people have, of course, been concerned with the problems examined in this series; but all too often this has been in individual or institutional isolation. These volumes will engage an international community that is large enough to develop research programmes and debates that will have enduring momentum and excitement.

Situated at the interface between museum, university and independent research institution, the series will address professional historians of science and technology, curators, those in charge of the day-to-day administration of museums and those who, so often passionately, simply enjoy visiting. As museums do in general, the series aims to build a bridge between historical research and the use and application of historical knowledge in education and the public understanding of science and technology.

Each volume will focus on a specific field of technology and science in its wider historical context. The first, and larger, part of each volume will present the honed products of presentation and debate at joint conferences. The second part will consist of exhibit reviews, critical expeditions into the respective museum's landscape, bibliographical overviews on recent literature, and the like.

The collaboration between three national institutions has been made possible by their directors. We thank Neil Cossons, Director of the Science Museum, Spencer Crew, Director of the National Museum of American History of the Smithsonian Institution, and Wolf Peter Fehlhammer, Director of the Deutsches Museum. Their personal enthusiasm for this project has made it possible.

Notes on contributors

Johannes Abele is completing his Ph.D. degree in the Program in History of Science and Technology at the Deutsches Museum, Munich. He studies the development of radiation measuring instruments in relation to the history of radiation safety. Since September 1997, he has been involved in a project at the Hannah-Arendt Institut für Totalitarismusforschung, Dresden, on the history of nuclear energy in the German Democratic Republic.

Ken Arnold is the Exhibitions Unit Manager at the Wellcome Trust, where he has worked since 1992. He also writes occasionally on the culture of museums past and present. He wrote his doctoral dissertation at Princeton on early-modern English cabinets of curiosities. Since then, he has worked in ethnographic, children's and historical museums.

Timothy M. Boon is Curator of Public Health at the Science Museum, London. He has recently completed his thesis *Health citizenship or health education? The health film in Britain, 1919–1945*.

Robert Bud is Curator of Biosciences and Head of Life and Communications Technologies at the Science Museum, London. Since 1994 he has also been responsible for collections-related research at the Museum. His speciality is the history of biotechnology.

Bernard Finn is curator of the electrical collections at the Smithsonian Institution's National Museum of American History where he has been responsible for more than two dozen exhibits, mostly dealing with electric power and communications. He has also written and lectured on the historical development of museums of science and technology. He holds a Ph.D. in the History of Science from the University of Wisconsin.

Patricia Peck Gossel is a curator in the Division of Science, Medicine, and Society at the Smithsonian Institution's National Museum of American History. Her interests include the history of the bacteriology laboratory, laboratory research instruments, and contraceptive technology.

Ghislaine Lawrence is Senior Curator of Clinical Medicine at the Science Museum, London. She was formerly a practising physician. Her research interests lie in the history of medical and surgical technologies, especially in the post-war era.

Kim Pelis holds a post-doctoral research fellowship jointly at the Science Museum and the Wellcome Institute in London. Her project is the history of blood transfusion. She holds a doctorate from Johns Hopkins University.

Helmuth Trischler is Head of the research department of the Deutsches Museum and Professor of History and History of Technology at the University of Munich.

Klaus Vogel studied cultural anthropology and education science in Tübingen, Germany. Since 1996, he has been Museum Director of the Deutsches Hygiene-Museum.

Robert Bud

Introduction

The revolution in the treatment of disease and injury that has taken place over the past two centuries is an urgent reality to patients and doctors alike; but, whereas change in medical theory and practice has made cure more likely and, in many cases, has reduced suffering, medicine embraces more than just techniques of treatment. Health and disease influence the lives and culture of everyone – including the robust citizen, as well as the sick and the medical profession – and frame the way we think of ourselves and run our daily lives.

Whereas, with its beauty and its distinctive features, the body is part of a person's identity, as a biological machine it is also a source of worry to its owner; daily life is replete with opportunities for medically defined "error" as we negotiate the issues of smoking, eating fatty food, exercise, polluting the air or taking pills at the right time. Professional lives, across the whole spectrum of modern economies, are now burdened with responsibilities for the "health and safety" of colleagues, newspaper readers puzzle over surrogate motherhood; cities encompass great hospitals and medical research centres that are held in some of the same awe as were cathedrals in former times. Meanwhile, the politics and economics of paying for medicine shape the debate over the future of the welfare state.

Such a multitude of connections are now being made by historians, museum curators and other commentators, that artefacts of medicine, also, are no longer to be seen merely in terms of their functional properties. Dissecting out the broader meaning can, nonetheless, present a considerable challenge of just the kind to which this series is directed. In this volume, five authors write about sets of artefacts, the origins of which range from the early nineteenth century to the late twentieth, and are today each to be found in museums: early blood transfusion apparatus, a plastic human replica, the Geiger counter, open-heart surgery equipment and packaging for the Pill.

The authors of each essay have been concerned about the broad significance of an artefact at the time of its innovation. Case by case, the use of the objects focuses attention not only on their medical purpose, but also on the meanings they held for all those who confronted them. As latter-day onlookers, we are therefore helped to see, not just machines, but also products of the imagination. The authors have also striven to show that those who today encounter the artefacts of this book, in its pages and even perhaps "in the flesh," will be confronting big subjects: blood, life, danger and conception.

For all the diversity of the topics, there are strong parallels between the accounts presented. It is striking that each artefact was the iconic focus of a story linking apparent opposites. Kim Pelis shows how blood transfusion apparatus developed by the London physician, James Blundell, in the 1820s was not just a technical device, it was seen by its "romantic" pioneer as mediating between life and death. This contemporary of Mary Shelley, the author of *Frankenstein*, and of Polidori, who wrote the first vampire romance, linked the "vital" qualities of blood to the apparently technical process of transfusion through a vision of the process of transfusion as bringing to life the virtually dead. "What is the meaning of my blood and my body?" is an ancient question that has continued to be reiterated – at never greater frequency than in the twentieth century. Strong feelings abide about blood transfusion. Scientific descriptions sit uncomfortably beside rich personal and, indeed, gory symbolism. Between the two has been the complex process of giving and getting blood.

The objectives of the proponents of the transparent man in the 1920s were the very opposite from those of the vitalists of a century earlier. For the successful businessman, Karl August Lindner, an advocate of organisation and education, the transparent models of human parts demonstrated, Klaus Vogel argues, how the human being exemplified an engineering system. Devised within the context of a new museum, The German Hygiene Museum in Dresden, the model known as the "Transparent Man" became an institutional, and indeed national symbol. Rather than the bloody process of dissecting a real human, transparent synthetic plastic enabled millions of visitors to the German Hygiene Museum and many other exhibitions to encounter the beautiful engineering of the "ideal" man and woman. Vogel demonstrates that this was both a successful technical product and a powerful ideological device, which has survived through four regimes since its birth in Weimar, Germany.

The Transparent Man was designed for the mass public; Ghislaine Lawrence has explored the meaning of a new technology for professional medical staff and the consequent shaping of a device. She examines the process of heart surgery under profound hypothermia devised between 1959 and 1961 by Charles Drew, a London surgeon. This technique converted the operating theatre into an engineering workshop: the heart rendered virtually bloodless and the equipment meeting precise design specifications, even if it proved too large to fit, in its entirety, into the operating theatre. Lawrence shows how even detailed design decisions made by Drew in concert with the designers and the process control engineers, APV – such as the selection of pneumatic rather than electronic controls – had their origins in process engineering practice. Thus this technology fitted a cultural space for the medical practitioners that was quite analogous to the space intended for the Transparent Man that was made from synthetic plastic.

The range of emotionally intense oppositions in medicine is, of course, not limited to the tension between gory body and engineering system. Johannes Abele's study of the Geiger counter shows how this device was used to separate safe environments from dangerous ones, in the workplace and in the aftermath of nuclear events. From the very time of the discovery of radioactivity, its accompanying threat was not susceptible to traditional concepts of safety. Even in its early days, the Geiger counter, invented in 1928 for purposes of scientific measurement, was also used for public display, and even before the Second World War, Geiger counters were used in hospitals to guarantee safety in the use of radium. After the war, the Gieger counter came to be portrayed as the key defence against new dangers posed by the nuclear power plant and the nuclear holocaust.

Finally, the packaging of the contraceptive pill is explored by Patricia Gossel. She finds its meaning in the space between the order and predictability of the laboratory allied to the discipline of the clinical trial on the one hand and, on the other, the disorder and unpredictability of daily life. Whereas historians have paid great attention to the Pill, they have, hitherto ignored both the packaging and its meaning. The focus on the development of compliance packaging therefore highlights the challenge of moving from abstract physiology to the daily lives of millions.

Our culture depends on the contrast between opposites, yet life is rarely so generous as to allow us to keep them entirely separate. Hospitals are places both of safety and of danger, the states of life and death can seem hardly separable. The authors here have located their subjects at such sensitive interfaces as between life and death, life and organisation, life and engineering, safety and danger, order and disorder. Each artefact has helped those encountering it to cope with the apparent confusion of categories, embodying or encapsulating stories that have been deeply reassuring. Blood, in the early nineteenth century, was seen to be a vital fluid that could actually bring to life one who was already dead, and the transfusor was designed to be an appropriate means by which this natural fluid should be handled. In the middle years of this century, in which the nature of man has been the subject of the most intense debate and has been caught up in ideologies that have wracked the western world, the Transparent Man and the technology of profound hypothermia seemed to reassure that living and engineering systems could be compared, however different they may appear. The Geiger counter and the Pill pack, by contrast, were means of distinguishing between the distinct states of safety and danger. While the accounts are rigorously historical, such issues are, of course, enduring.

Encounters with such devices today can often be powerful and moving experiences that engage the viewer's concerns not only with the culture of the past, but also with the dilemmas of the present. Medical museums exhibiting their collections have this twofold quality of historicity and relevance. Research on the material culture of medicine has, in general, been based in museums; the way in which these institutions represent artefacts and material culture defines our culture's attitudes.

Two review papers in this volume reflect on museums at various levels of generality, linking their objectives, exhibits and collections. A very specific approach was taken to the reviews, for there are many possible aspects of visitor care and interaction that go beyond the boundaries of this book. Instead of looking at every possible aspect, these review articles focus upon the problem of telling a meaningful history through objects and exhibits.

In his study of the Science Museum, Tim Boon, one of the curators responsible for *Health Matters*, which opened at the Science Museum in 1994, reports on that gallery and on a series of more recent temporary exhibitions. He reflects on the place of *Health Matters* in the development of the Museum's presentation of history, and describes the exhibit section by section.

Ken Arnold reviews the world's medical museums, linking the institutions' histories, their collections and their exhibits. He advocates treating the museums themselves as historic artefacts. They can thus be treated in the same way as other authors have dealt with individual instruments. He reports upon more than 50 institutions, surveying the landscape of the medical museum world, and reflecting on the kinds of medical history it portrays. He asks for more temporary exhibitions with thematic cross-disciplinary approaches that bring together science, technology and art and thereby widen the horizon of history.

With the other authors of this volume, Arnold believes that these institutions should strive not just to make the objects within them audible, but even to make them sing!

Kim Pelis

Transfusion, with teeth

Indigo: "He's dead! He can't talk!"
Miracle Max: "Look who knows so much! Well, it just so happens that your friend here is only mostly dead. There's a big difference between mostly dead and all dead ... Mostly dead is slightly alive. Now all dead, with all dead there's only one thing you can do."
Indigo: "What's that?"
Max: "Go through their clothes and look for loose change."
– The Princess Bride

When respiration is once stopped, she is gone beyond the reach of known remedy, under received methods of management – not even transfusion itself can save her; – a solemn pause follows, presently broken by ejaculations scarcely audible; some dear friend sobbing and in tears, exclaims, "Can you do nothing? Is there no hope?"
– James Blundell, 1827[1]

In 1818, London accoucheur[2] and physiologist, James Blundell, suggested that persons dying of haemorrhage might be saved by the timely transfusion of blood from a willing human donor. Although his first trial, conducted later that same year, was on a man dying from an ulcer, Blundell soon became convinced that the procedure should be limited to women on the verge of death from uterine haemorrhage. Here, he believed, transfusion held great therapeutic promise. Through the 1820s and 1830s, a small group of British accoucheurs carried out transfusions on such women, publishing accounts of their efforts – many of them apparently successful – in medical journals such as the controversial *Lancet*. Successful case histories often told of how such women were veritably re-animated by transfused blood. By 1825, the potential of transfusion had become the subject of intense debate in British medical circles.[3]

Blundell himself provided two suggestions of how he came to think of the movement of blood between bodies as potentially therapeutic. First were the animal transfusion experiments of fellow Edinburgh medical school alumnus, John Leacock (1816), and second was the sympathy he felt for haemorrhaging women.[4] Certainly, both of these factors encouraged the young accoucheur's thinking. Yet, in 1818, transfusion was in its second century of prohibition, having been banned from medical practice after the death of a recipient in 1667.[5] Moreover, blood-letting was still seen as a therapeutic procedure, which could even be used to *treat* uterine haemorrhage. How, then, did Blundell come to think of blood's transfusion as therapeutic? The question centres on the nature of a medical innovation;

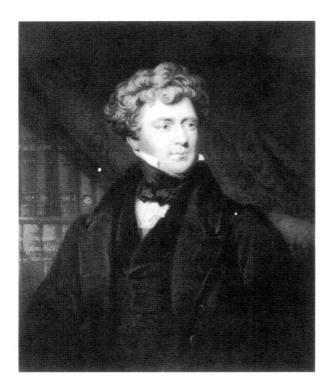

Figure 1. James Blundell. Stipple engraving by J. Cochran after H. Room.

its answer may be found in the culture in which transfusion was devised. Culture conventionally refers to ideas, ideologies and institutions; I wish to highlight, too, the material culture of instruments devised to move blood between bodies.

Many members of the early nineteenth-century British cultural elite were concerned with the significance of the dramatic changes that had accompanied the close of the eighteenth century. Revolutions in French politics and chemistry, physiological discoveries of resuscitation and galvanism – all suggested that the natural order might be revealed, dismantled and reassembled.[6] Such concerns, and their possibilities, fed the imaginations of a genre of writers loosely dubbed "the Romantics."[7] Further, they inspired elite medical practitioners, intent on distancing themselves from "lesser" healers in the active "medical market place," to devise a Romantic professional self-image: that of the lone creative genius, obsessed by his search for truth to penetrate uncharted territories and "unveil" nature.[8]

Perhaps the central "uncharted territory" concerning these Romantically-inclined medical elite was death itself. Resuscitation and galvanism helped open a conceptual space between life and death that was ideally suited for definition by medical authority.[9] Known as "apparent death," this space encouraged these practitioners to take on a new, interventionist role at the death-bed, as it charged their aspirations for professional power. Porter and Porter have dubbed these aspirations "medical promethianism."[10] This conceptual and professional nexus, I shall argue, also expressed itself in the more technologically concrete form of blood transfusion. On the most general level, then, Blundell's innovation may be read as a Romantic re-animation of the apparently dead.

Accompanying this general reading is the more specific, if more abstract, connection of transfusion to two mythic figures of Gothic romance. For, in 1818, the very year that Blundell introduced his transfusion, Frankenstein's monster was "born;" and, in 1819, the vampire was introduced to polite literary society.[11] The monster and the vampire are on one level images of Romantic genius gone awry – attempts to control life instead turning into forces of evil.[12] Upon examining parallels between the substance of blood and electricity, and the form of the instrumental manipulation of vital forces, one may also understand transfusion as the Romantic end of a continuum with the Gothic. Transfusion is the heroic channelling of the vital principle: the monster, the evil potential inherent in an act of such hubris.

There is yet another, related, reading of transfusion that relies upon more specific elements of medical self-definition and Romantic imagination. Blundell, a licensed physician, was not only a practising man-midwife, but also one of England's most popular obstetrical lecturers. Much has been made by medical historians of forceps and the man-midwife's rise to power. With Blundell's transfusion, the medically trained man-midwife gained further justification for a prominent place in the birthing chamber. In a sense, then, one might present transfusion as an obstetrician's efforts to control the potentially fatal effects of uterine haemorrhage, and thereby play midwife to the rebirth of the birthing mother.[13]

I hope to show that all three of these readings help illuminate the medical innovation of human-to-human transfusion.

Such an interpretation must necessarily approach the topic from numerous angles. Thus I will begin with the story of Blundell's life and transfusion work, told as a kind of "historical fiction" in the voice of a plausible character – a former student of Blundell's. This stylised narrative voice is in fact composed from a chorus of Blundell's champions, including his most vocal advocate, Charles Waller.[14] I have chosen this unconventional approach to underscore how easily the historical facts of Blundell's work fit into patterns then characteristic of the Romantic (medical) genius.

The historical backdrop for the transfusion story is constructed from recent scholarship on late eighteenth- and early nineteenth-century ideas and practices surrounding re-animation and Romanticism.[15] My argument goes through four stages to reach its conclusion. First, I will provide a brief summary of the re-animating strands of scientific thought current around 1818. Second, I will review the medical applications of "re-animation" and the related construction of a Romantic professional self-image by British medical elite. Within this section, I will also examine Blundell's exposure to these ideas, both scientific and Romantic, during his medical education at Edinburgh and in London. Third, I will follow them into Gothic literature. Initially, this excursion will take us into their well-studied realm of expression in Mary Shelley's *Frankenstein*; from here, I shall attempt to move them towards the vampiric, as articulated in Polidori's "The Vampyre." My argument will be drawn in part from conceived similarities between blood and electricity. Finally, I will examine blood transfusion within this framework. I shall add descriptions of transfused women that at once resonate with corpses and vampiric victims, reflect a vitalistic conception of blood as re-animating fluid, and support an argument for transfusion *apparatus* as the final link between transfusion and Romantic re-animation.

***

James Blundell: A Romance?

September, 1834

I write, dear Brother, with the sad news that my teacher and friend, Dr James Blundell, will be leaving Guy's Hospital, to teach – he swears it – no more.[16] I know you have been diligently preparing to join me here in London so as to learn from the Master – indeed, that your arrival is imminent – and so I must regretfully suggest that you follow your original plan. Meet me here in a year's time. We should both be in a better situation, and I shall have had time to find a new guide for your medical studies.

October, 1834

Dear Eddy,

Indeed, I shall be happy to tell you more of our Blundell. I have enticed you to leave Edinburgh and join me here with only the vaguest references to his physiological teachings and surgical innovations. Now, I may elaborate upon these and reveal other qualities he possesses – qualities that I believed would appeal to you even as they did to me.[17]

First, some background. Blundell was born here in London in December of 1790. The quality of the classical education given him by the Rev. Thomas Thomason is evident to anyone fortunate enough to have heard him speak. Following in the path of his beloved uncle, John Haighton, Blundell studied "at the Southwark united hospitals of St. Thomas and Guy's, where he had for teachers Sir Astley Cooper and Mr. Cline,"[18] as well as Haighton himself. You have certainly heard tell of Haighton's contributions to obstetricy and of his controversial physiological experiments – for which some have dubbed him "the Merciless Doctor."[19] Apparently, his nephew has not been deterred by such criticisms, as he has since unflinchingly supported animal experimentation conducted in the service of physiological inquiry. His hospital training completed, Blundell went to our own town's medical school – Edinburgh University, where he took his degree in 1813. Returning thereupon to London, and to Guy's and St Thomas's, he assisted his uncle with his teaching duties – succeeding Haighton as "Lecturer upon Physiology and Midwifery" in 1818. To my knowledge, he has never been married, remaining instead wholly committed to his science.

James Blundell always drew a crowd, whether to his obstetrical or to his physiological lectures. Perhaps it was in part the legacy of being Haighton's nephew. Perhaps the crowds came because of his oratorical skills. An apt classical reference or Latin phrase would often provide the eloquent edge of a cutting remark he would wield to expose the absurdities of many an accepted – but untested – medical assumption.[20] Then again, it may have been the evident joy with which he challenged the medical profession to go beyond its standard practices and into forbidden realms such as blood transfusion and abdominal surgery. He is certainly one of a very few men in England teaching physiology and reporting unapologetically on animal experiments – and has as such drawn the acclaim and the wrath of medical journals and societies alike. James Blundell is indeed a rare kind of man – a creative genius, passionate in his pursuit of truth.[21]

In his lectures, "Dr. Blundell soars to the loftiest regions of romantic impossibility."[22] Never shall I forget his inspiring charge:

Can a man have his abdomen laid open and recover? Physiology teaches us that he may. Can life be restored when the patient is dying from bleeding, by the transfusion of new blood into the veins? Physiology teaches us that it has been so restored. Can a fourth part of the human body be cut away, by the amputation of the thigh at the hip joint, and the expanse of wounded surface heal by the first intention? Physiology teaches us that it may. This is the crown of physiology; – by putting us in possession of the powers of natural bodies, by reading us a lecture, as it were, on the jurisprudence by which those powers are regulated, and by thus making us acquainted with those laws and powers, she enables us, to a certain extent, to mould the material world at our pleasure, and to work on natural bodies at our will. Realising, in some degree, the tales of romance, she leads us, like Vathek, into the intimate recesses of nature, and puts into our hands the talismans by which her operations are controlled.[23]

What possibilities his words opened to my mind! Might we, I wondered, unveil nature and direct its power? On that same day, I resolved to learn the science of physiology, to use it to push back the tide of death and restore life. We might even control the vital principle. This is precisely what I knew Blundell to have done. Indeed, I was witness to it. And, as I know you share my deep interest in the possibilities inherent in the transfusion of human blood, I shall tell you more of Blundell's investigations.

Transfusion, although an old – even ancient – idea, rests on new knowledge that experimental study has provided us, into the nature of death and the role of the blood in the body. "We know," Blundell has explained, "that in hanging or submersion, death, at first, is apparent only, and not real; for a certain period after respiration stops, resuscitation is still possible. Now, that death from bleeding may also for a time be apparent, is by no means unlikely; and it is not impossible, therefore, that transfusion may be of service, if performed within a given period even after the breathing has been stopped."[24] The blood's "passive vitality" provides a kind of galvanising force that we are now able to marshal to serve our re-animating desires.[25] Taken from a member of the same species – and preferably from a male of the species, as men "bleed more freely and are less liable to faint"[26] – and injected slowly into women "apparently dead" of haemorrhage, the blood has the power to restore life itself.

Blundell often commented on how it was sympathy that had first compelled him to use transfused blood in an effort to restore life to women sinking under uterine haemorrhage. Yet, only when I first attended such a woman did I understand what he meant.[27] By the time I was summoned to her bedside, "she resembled a person actually dead."[28] My examination showed, however, that some life remained. "The countenance of the patient ... was completely blanched, not the least appearance of redness being observable in the cheeks or lips, the extremities cold, the breathing very laborious, the pulse excessively feeble, the whole surface of the body was cool, and the skin had a soft yielding feel, and indeed her general appearance was that of a woman sinking from exhaustion."[29] Immediately, I sent for her husband, and for Blundell.

By the time Blundell arrived with his "Gravitator" transfusion device, the small room was quite crowded. I was instructed to prepare "the husband, a hearty coal-heaver,"[30] for venesection, as Blundell attended the patient and set up his equipment. The apparatus itself was quite a marvel: it consisted of a cup into which the husband was to be bled (*see* Figure 2). This cup was attached atop a long brass tube, or staff, that allowed blood to flow by the force of gravity into a cannula more than a foot below. A band firmly attached the cannula to the woman's arm, and a vice, affixed to a nearby chair, provided support to the whole of the system. Blundell explained that he had designed his Gravitator so that the blood retained its vital powers as it moved from vein to vein (an unnatural, but necessary, circuit) through the metal.[31] Animal tests, he assured us, had long since convinced him that the artificial materials themselves would not make the blood unfit for passage.[32]

The equipment, donor and patient prepared, we proceeded with the operation. "Two ounces of that fluid were drawn from the arm of the patient's husband ... and transferred to her. The result was surprising, the patient immediately opened her eyes, which had been shut, and the pulse became sensible; the extremities recovered a little heat, and the countenance improved."[33] We then provided her with stimulants. When she later declined, we repeated the procedure, throwing in another "two ounces and a half from the arm of the woman's husband." The result was astonishing: "life seemed to be immediately reanimated as by an electric spark."[34] It shall perhaps come as no surprise to you, dear brother, if I confess this to

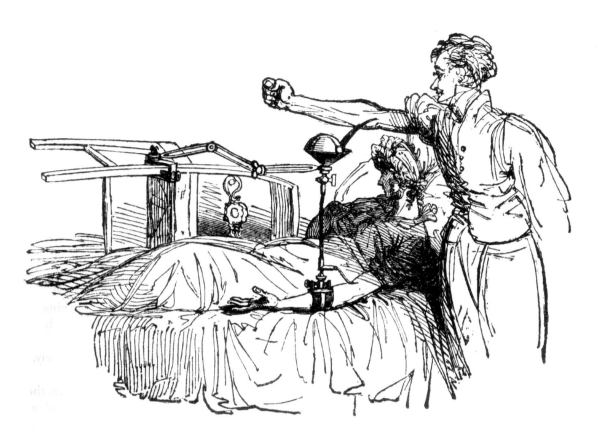

Figure 2. Blundell's Gravitator in use. Arguably the most famous image of transfusion's history in nineteenth-century Britain (from James Blundell, "Observations on Transfusion of Blood, with a Description of his Gravitator," The Lancet 2 [1828–29]: 321–24).

have been "the most gratifying case that has ever rewarded my professional solicitude."[35]

I make this assertion with the deepest possible conviction: "the profession and the public at large are under deep and lasting obligations to Dr. James Blundell;" his name shall be handed down "to posterity, as one of the greatest benefactors of *womankind.*" Not all, however, have seen the genius of his contributions, and have, out of ignorance or jealousy, instead treated his work "with neglect, opposition, and ridicule, still he was not to be deterred from his purpose till the remedy had experienced a fair trial."[36] Indeed, members of the Medical Society of London, and even editors of certain medical journals (chief among these the editor of the *Medical Repository*, "generalissimo of the opposers of his operation"), have allied themselves in resistance to Blundell's work; and, were it not for staunch supporters such as the editor of *The Lancet*, I fear our cause would long ago have been lost.[37] I am particularly at a loss to explain how a profession so recently under attack for purchasing "resurrected" corpses for medical study could so easily dismiss a procedure that gives it the power to steal back life from death itself. Thus it is with some dread that I witness my teacher quit his position, as his untimely departure will leave the operation of transfusion, still in its infancy, an orphan.

I hope, upon my return to Edinburgh at Christmas, to have final news concerning possibilities for your education. Meanwhile, I send a gift – a slim volume, penned by another Edinburgh medical graduate, John Polidori. It is called *The Vampyre*, and is much in the Byronic spirit of which we are both so fond. Meanwhile, I remain,

     Yours,

     C.

***

The structure of this particular historical fiction is borrowed with little shame (if less poetry) from the first section of *Frankenstein*. It has been applied to underscore the close fit between Blundell's life story and transfusion work and the narrative structures of Gothic romance. Blundell is presented, both in autobiographical asides and by his followers, as a solitary genius, driven by his quest to unveil nature, and ostracised by society as a result. In short, his is the story of the Romantic hero who, examined from a slightly different angle, shades into the Gothic. Before turning to a discussion of the significance of these correlations for medicine generally and transfusion in particular, it is necessary to examine the scientific work that encouraged their emergence.

Apparently Dead

How do we recognise death? More specifically, how can we differentiate between someone who appears to be dead, and someone who really *is* dead? To say that an incorrect judgement would bring about *unfortunate* consequences is perhaps the extreme of understatement. The fear of premature burial is ancient and profound; it has been tied to a host of funeral rituals and folk tales – including the myth of the undead, or the vampire.[38] At the historical moment of the reintroduction of transfusion to medical practice, life and the body were undergoing studies that had profound consequences for the perception of the line separating life and death. The guiding question seemed to be not so much where to find a pre-existing line between life and death, but rather, whether experimental knowledge now had the power to determine where it was to be drawn.[39] Resuscitation, galvanism and physiology all had formative consequences for the rising medical significance of apparent death.[40]

The formation of Humane Societies throughout the Continent and Great Britain from 1767 onwards had drawn great attention to the phenomenon of apparent death. These societies focused on the prevention of premature burial and the resuscitation of the drowned – and disseminated this information to the public. It was a trio of medical men – Thomas Cogan (accoucheur), William Hawes (apothecary) and J. C. Lettsom (physician) – who applied these ideas in London, establishing a Humane Society there in 1774. To draw attention to their cause, members of the Humane Society (which became "Royal" in 1790) distributed leaflets to the public, offered rewards to those who managed to resuscitate drowning victims, and even attracted members of the clergy, persuading them to preach the gospel of resuscitation in their churches. Their efforts did not go unrewarded. Membership swelled and branches of the Royal Humane Society [RHS] were established throughout Britain.[41] The concept of apparent death was increasingly coupled in the public mind with the possibility of its reversal – doing little to harm the reputation of medicine. The RHS's resuscitating *methods* were also well publicised on posters and leaflets and pulpits. For only by familiarity with these methods could members of the public be expected to reach into icy waters and re-animate apparently dead bodies.[42] Briefly, initial advice was that one was to carry the body flat, warm it, apply stimulants – including rubbing and enemas – and, with the first signs of life, administer brandy. Blood-letting, too, was initially advocated, but quickly abandoned.[43] In an effort to update these methods in accordance with the latest medical knowledge, the Society solicited essays on apparent death by arranging competitions. A winning essay of 1795, by A. Fothergill, explored possible applications of medical electricity to the purposes of resuscitation.[44]

Electricity had been much in vogue in the eighteenth century, as Leyden jars shocked salon-goers throughout Britain and Europe.[45] With the work of Luigi Galvani, however, the movement of electricity through living bodies took on new scientific respectability. His famous studies on animal electricity, dating from the 1780s until his death in 1798, investigated the nature of the "nervous fluid" that appeared to stimulate the movement of living bodies. The interpretations he gave to his stimulated and jumping frogs' legs drew the criticism of Allesandro Volta, thus setting up their duelling experiments of the 1790s. In addition to "galvanism's" extension of electricity into physiological realms, it also brought current electricity to bear on the public imagination. For, upon Galvani's death, his nephew, Giovanni Aldini, attempted to win his uncle's case by popularising it. Accordingly, he animated severed calves' heads and hanged criminals' bodies before numerous audiences.[46] When Aldini brought his travelling electrical show to London, he brought it to the Royal Humane Society.[47]

Across the Channel, French physicians were exploring the consequences of political revolutionary upheaval in the reorganisation of medical structures that facilitated pathological correlation and the rise of the "Paris Clinical School."[48] If resultant therapies were few, future possibilities seemed limitless. It was the famous French clinician and pioneer of tissue pathology, Xavier Bichat, who at this time articulated his famous definition of "life" as those forces that oppose death. Similarly, a younger member of this group, François Magendie, was testing the line between life and death through extensive animal experimentation. Physiological experimentation on animals was less formally developed in Britain than in France; however, it did exist. John Haighton, Blundell's uncle, conducted vivisections on rabbits to test his theories about generation (*see* Figure 3). A group of like-minded British medical men, including Humphry Davy and Benjamin Brodie, participated in the "Animal Chemistry Club," where they discussed the consequences of physiological and chemical investigations on the nature of life.[49]

At the same time, a renewed interest in vitalism became evident in the thinking of medical elites. Indeed, Edinburgh University had a strong tradition of commitment to a vitalistic view of the body centring upon the nervous system, which dated from the mid eighteenth century. The medical school's influential teacher, William Cullen, had espoused a system in which the "nervous fluid" possessed a power "unique to life," and was responsible for the body's "sensibility" and its integrating "sympathy."[50] Similarly, blood was believed by some to be a likely container for the vital principle. The status of blood as a "vital fluid," although changing in details over time, had remained a fundamental assumption of Western thought since at least the beginning of its recorded existence.[51] Even William Harvey, in his pioneering studies establishing the blood's circulation in the body, had remained reverential in his attitudes towards blood.[52] Enlightenment studies may have provided insight into oxygen and its role in the blood; nevertheless, this was not enough to effect a wholesale movement away from a perception of the vitality of blood. The famous eighteenth-century British surgeon and philosophical speculator on life, John Hunter, was committed to a vitalistic conception of blood in which its coagulation led to tissue formation.[53] As manifested in physiological inquiry, early nineteenth-century vitalism no longer considered the life principle to be a kind of "seat of the soul." Owsei Temkin has traced the changing definition of vitalism, from the sensualism of the Scottish Enlightenment to the "vital materialism" of early nineteenth-century physiology. As is evident in the interpretive assumptions of Magendie and others, vital materialism located any potential "vital principle" in the material of the living body.[54] While this position was not purely reductionistic, it did alienate those who espoused a strict Cartesian dualism and the separate existence of a rational soul. Notwithstanding, "vital materialism" left open the working analogy between blood, electricity and life. In the 1820s, Edinburgh medical graduate Jean-Louis Prevost, with his collaborator Jean-Baptiste Dumas, applied galvanic currents to blood in order to discern how the blood formed tissue and to confirm their own "globular" notions of blood.[55] Marshall Hall, another Edinburgh graduate and contemporary of Blundell, explored the relationship between nervous and circulatory systems in a series of physiological experiments.[56]

In an event that Marilyn Butler has tied directly to the imaginative foundations of *Frankenstein*, vitalism spilled from medical discourse into public debate. In 1814, John Abernethy, President of the Royal College of Surgeons, delivered the Hunterian lecture on the "vital principle," which he believed – he claimed, with Hunter – was added to the body, much like a soul. It was not contained within the material of the body itself. His claims drew the intellectual fire of his student, William Lawrence, who asserted that Hunter would have instead supported *him* in his more materialistic view that the vital principle, such as it is, resides in matter itself. Lawrence was to become the Shelleys' physician and, Butler persuasively argues, his vitalistic debate with Abernethy helped inspire Mary Shelley's vision of Victor Frankenstein.[57] Medical men with strong opinions about vitalism and re-animation linked literary and experimental realms.

Clearly, the nexus of blood and galvanic currents, of tissues and nerves – of these potential bearers of integrating vital fluids – was assumed to be a tight one, and was studied by some physiologists in this spirit. This nexus, as we shall see, also encouraged elite British medical practitioners to aspire to the colonisation of new territories, both professional and intellectual. It also provided the cultural environment in which James Blundell was raised.

"Unveilers of Nature"

In a recent article, Ludmilla Jordanova has described Mary Shelley's famous experimenter, Victor Frankenstein, as the embodiment of qualities that characterised the ideals of early nineteenth-century British medical elite: reclusive, passionate, thirsty for knowledge (although perpetually

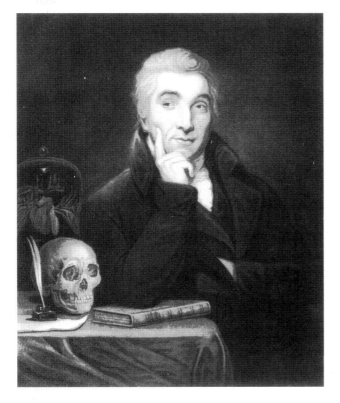

Figure 3. John Haighton and the icons of a Romantic medical practitioner. Mezzotint by I. Kennerly, 1818.

unsatisfied in attempts to attain it), drawn to things "marginal, contentious or on the boundaries of what could be controlled."[58] It is precisely these qualities, she argues, that elite medical practitioners were drawing upon in an effort to create a powerful, persuasive and coherent professional identity. Jordanova refers to the medical quest to blaze uncharted intellectual territories as "unveiling nature;" to the identity that medical men were constructing, she attaches the label "Romantic." The connection of these medical men to Shelley's Frankenstein is described as a kind of continuum, which shades from the Romantic (espoused by the medics) to the Gothic (embodied by Frankenstein).[59] In a sense, these extremes are linked in the fashion of the normal and the pathological. The link itself is the quest to unveil nature, and the kinds of knowledge this quest might reveal.[60]

The Romanticising medical elite was particularly fond of coupling its professional aspirations with power over death. It is generally accepted that the sciences I have loosely referred to as "re-animating" – resuscitation, galvanism, aspects of physiology – were important to Romantic thinkers, both literary and scientific.[61] The knowledge they uncovered, as we have seen, opened up the space between life and death. Within this space, "apparent death" increasingly became a place of promise, where medical intervention might be possible.[62] For medical men, who were at this time actively competing for dominance in what has been called a teeming "marketplace" of healers, and who traditionally had no professional role at the death-bed, Romantic control over apparent death offered both a new potency and a new place. As Jordanova argues, even if these medical men could as yet *do* little more to stave off death than could their predecessors, the possibility that they *might*, could be channelled into a professional image that effectively increased their power.[63]

Before moving forward to a discussion about Blundell's place within this group of "Romantic unveilers of nature," it is necessary to qualify my use of the loaded but useful term "Romantic." First, the group we now call "Romantic" did not, in fact, apply the term to themselves – it is rather a term conferred upon them by history.[64] Temporally, the Romantics may be traced back to the 1740s and forward into the 1820s; nationally, they appeared throughout Europe, Britain and even the nascent USA. Within these differences in time and place, they embraced different ideas and ideologies.[65] They also spanned intellectual disciplines in a way that characterised the fluidity of disciplinary boundaries at that time. In David Knight's words, "one cannot define members of the Romantic Movement as one might members of a political party ... almost everybody was, in some degree [a Romantic]."[66]

How, then, am I using the term "Romanticism"? Both in its broadest and in its most specific sense. Broadly, we still use the term to describe individuals society considers to be solitary "geniuses." Heroic portrayals of brilliant but misunderstood artists and scientists, possessed by a unique vision that allows them to uncover or "create" something new, and set on the margins of society in consequence, are common themes of popular cinema and literature.[67] Our culture remains committed to a view of these solitary individuals as the leaders of true social and intellectual change.

At the same time, early nineteenth-century Britain was developing its own form of Romanticism. Most closely identified with Lord Byron and Percy Shelley, this focused on classicism, the secular study of myth and religion, and condemned the evils of despotic and over-extended governments.[68] In short, this particular Romanticism championed individual, creative thought and romanticised foreign cultures with characteristic "orientalism."[69] "The unknown" was there to feed the imagination and provoke exploration – impulses fuelled by the Romantic fascination with scientific knowledge, and particularly with the works of Erasmus Darwin, who had himself suggested the possibilities of transfusion.[70]

Surrounded by images of death and vivisected animals, John Haighton was a veritable archetype of the Romantic medical unveiler. As we have seen, Haighton essentially raised his sister's son, James Blundell, and trained him to follow in his professional footsteps. Medical Romantics such as Sir Astley Cooper extended Blundell's medical training in London, before he was sent off to formal study for his MD at Edinburgh University, "home of Cullen's nervous vitalism." Blundell's education was one in which the line between the quick and the dead was continually being redrawn by medical intervention, with resuscitation stressed alongside nervous integration.[71] Blundell himself had studied medical jurisprudence and learned in detail the methods of differentiating apparent from real death.[72]

The re-animating potential of medicine was the subject of several dissertations at the medical school of Edinburgh University in the decades surrounding Blundell's study there. One such dissertation, written by John Davies (a member of Blundell's graduating class of 1813) reviewed a range of apparent deaths, brought about by submersion, strangulation or electrical shock, and possible re-animating techniques.[73] Blundell himself, perhaps influenced by Edinburgh's nervous orientation, and certainly encouraged by his uncle Haighton's physiological perspective, wrote his dissertation on the differences between the senses employed for hearing speech and hearing music.[74]

Indeed, at this same time, the sensible citizens of Edinburgh, perhaps conversant with methods of resuscitating the drowned and the applications of galvanism, were going to great lengths to ensure that the bodies Blundell and his colleagues dissected to obtain this medical knowledge would not be their own. For this was also the time when the body-snatching escapades of the "resurrectionists" were adding a new fear to the host of old fears surrounding burial: that of being stolen from out of the grave and sold to medical men, to be dissected like a common criminal.[75] Burke and Hare had yet to be caught; nevertheless, grave-robbing was notorious enough for the wealthy to invest in structures that would ensure their undisturbed eternal rest.[76] In what seems almost an ironic reversal of the resuscitating ideals of the Humane Societies, some body-snatchers treated the old, infirm or vagrant *as* apparently dead, hastening their real deaths with suffocation in order to collect pay for their corpses.[77] In this context of grave-robbing, re-animation and growing medical power over the body, it is little wonder that Gothic and Romantic tales captured the imaginations of so many.

In essence, James Blundell was steeped in the Romantic professional aspirations of his time. He represents a second generation of British medical elite to hold these ideals and, as such, perhaps held them less self-consciously than did the first generation, which had articulated them. An avid supporter of individual thought and of creative genius, Blundell's epithet could well have been, "think for yourself." In physiology lectures, he classified men as being of two types. The first type appropriated and applied received knowledge – an important task. The second type, however, were "men of vigorous power, capable of thinking for themselves, fond of thinking for themselves – men who take more pleasure in the operation of the intellect than in the Circean styles of sensuality." To such men, who "make incursions into unknown regions, and subjugate, as it were, fresh territories of the intellectual world," the demi-gods of the human species, the connecting link between man and superior intelligences, Blundell held forth physiological knowledge as the key to power over nature.[78]

Further, Blundell compared the physiologist's aspirations to the penetrating adventures of Vathek. Vathek is the main character in William Beckford's 1786 "oriental tale," in which Caliph Vathek descends into hell in his quest for forbidden knowledge.[79] This quest necessarily entails the sacrifice of more than a few lives; the story itself influenced many a Romantic writer, in addition to Blundell.[80] *The Lancet* twice described Blundell's "personal appearances" at social functions, and in both, Blundell struck an "oriental" pose. At the first, he delivered the aforementioned "soaring romantic" speech in which he spoke of the "sun of medicine, sinking into the western hemisphere, to be soon plunged for ever into the interminable empire of darkness," and of "pyramids, that survive the wreck of time, and smile amidst surrounding desolation."[81] Shortly thereafter, he is described as appearing at a costume party dressed as a "turban'd turk."[82] Clearly, Blundell adopted both the style and the content of Romantic critiques then being levelled against a West that ignored the mysterious potential of "oriental" cultures.

In addition, Blundell cited many a Latin verse and Greek mythical or philosophical example, even in formulating his own life's struggles. Shortly before he left Guy's Hospital, for example, he compared his plight to that of a famous Greek seeker of truth: "Notwithstanding the sneers of his comic countryman, who placed him among the clouds, it was the just boast of Socrates, that he had brought down philosophy from her airy speculations, into the commerce of mankind."[83] He saw himself as having attempted to do the same with physiology: "If I have myself any claim, however small, to rank among the supporters of transfusion, it lies entirely in this: that, undeterred by clamour or scepticism, I have made it my endeavour, again, to bring the operation into notice." With Vathek and Frankenstein (and even Faust himself), James Blundell sought to penetrate the veil of nature, behind which he hoped to expose blood and reveal the cavities of the body. He, too, felt that the world turned against him when he succeeded in so doing.

Although he was not directly so, Blundell could well have been the model for Victor Frankenstein. For, up until the moment Blundell quit his job and walked permanently away from his experimental crusade, his life's story fits strikingly into those narrative structures. Like Victor Frankenstein, James Blundell was a solitary man obsessed by a vision of controlling nature – even eschewing romantic contact of "the other sort" while so doing.[84] Before turning finally to a contextual interpretation of Blundell's transfusion work, then, it is necessary to say a bit more about the twin anti-heroes of Gothic romance: Frankenstein's monster and "The Vampyre."

Romancing the Vampire

The story of the night that conceived modernity's most influential monster myths – Frankenstein's monster and the vampire – is both famous and contested.[85] It is known to have taken place at Lake Geneva in mid June 1816 among Percy Shelley, Mary Godwin, Lord Byron and Byron's physician, John Polidori. Apparently, Byron suggested that each of the assembled individuals devise a ghost story – a challenge that *eventually* gave rise to Mary Shelley's *Frankenstein* and Polidori's "The Vampyre."[86] At some point either immediately before or after Byron issued his challenge, Shelley, a long-time devotee of the natural sciences, had been discussing the finer points of galvanism and the possibilities of re-animating the dead. While it is evident from Polidori's diary that he and Shelley had engaged in such a conversation, it is unclear whether Shelley's partner in this particular conversation, to which Mary Godwin was a silent witness, was Byron – as Godwin herself later remembered it – or Polidori. Polidori, a recent medical graduate of Edinburgh University, would have been well versed in medical electricity and its uses, as a result of his education and of his membership of Edinburgh's famous debating society, the Speculative Society.[87] Regardless of the discussant's identity, Godwin was greatly impressed with the potential powers of electricity, later attributing the inspiration for her popular novel to this discussion.

It is to *Frankenstein* that I first turn. In Mary Shelley's work, one may see the wedding of efforts to control nature to a general cultural angst over the post-Revolutionary dismemberment of the body politic and over the more concrete dismemberment of resurrected bodies.[88] The result is a kind of corpse, stitched together and re-animated through the applications of experimental knowledge. At one point, Victor Frankenstein describes the desire that moved him toward creating his monster: "I entered with the greatest diligence into the search of ... the elixir of life ... Wealth was an inferior object; but what glory would attend the discovery, if I could banish disease from the human frame and render man invulnerable to any but a violent death!" He then proceeds to describe a thunderstorm he had witnessed, in which an old oak tree was struck by lightening and "reduced to thin ribbons of wood" – thereby introducing to his already-charged mind the powers of electricity.[89] Finally, into this primordial scientific soup, Frankenstein adds University study of chemistry and physiology: "After days and nights of incredible labour and fatigue, I succeeded in discovering the cause of generation and life; nay, more, I became myself capable of bestowing animation upon lifeless matter."[90]

Subsequently, Frankenstein invades the "dissecting room and the slaughter-house" in his quest to "renew life where death had apparently devoted the body to corruption."[91] The pieces collected and assembled, a feverishly obsessed Victor "collected the instruments of life around me, that I might infuse a spark of being into the lifeless thing that lay at my feet."[92] Unlike the film versions that followed a century later, the book gives no account of exactly what these "instruments of life" were, or how they might have been used. Instead, Shelley leaves our imaginations to fill in details from the hints Victor has dropped of physiology, chemistry and splintered oaks. That these instruments were effective is evident as the "lifeless thing" comes to life – ultimately to effect the demise of its creator.

Let us examine Victor Frankenstein's work as it fits into the Romantic definition of creativity. James Twitchell has recently offered the following synthesis:

For the Romantic artist this [creative] "process" usually involves four relatively stable parts: the artist, the audience, the object of art (artefact) and the subject of art. Creation at its simplest involves the movement of energy (life, imagination, attention) from one part to another. Although individual Romantic artists believed the process worked in different ways, they agreed that when art succeeded, the resultant energy in the system was greater than the initial charge.[93]

While Twitchell is applying this argument to the vampiric, it can equally well be applied to Frankenstein. Victor has sacrificed his own vital force (his declining health and feverish state are often alluded to, both as he creates the monster, and as he later pursues it), and he has supplied a powerful current of energy to animate the dead. His monster is at once "object of art" and product of an experimental science that has successfully understood, and thereby controlled, nature. The "forces opposing death" have redrawn the boundaries of life.

Such creative movement of energy is precisely the dynamic of the vampiric relationship – and, like Frankenstein's monster, the thing created is a kind of dark life force. Not coincidentally, the vampire made his move from folk tales to literature through the pen of another member of that small Romantic gathering at Lake Geneva: Dr John Polidori. Polidori, a precocious recent graduate of Edinburgh medical faculty, had by the time of this June evening, fallen out with his employer. Borrowing from a story fragment articulated by Byron himself, Polidori fleshed out a brief tale that introduced the aristocratic, amoral and life-draining vampire, Lord Ruthven, and a handsome and precocious young man "of high romantic feeling," Aubrey.[94] Little imagination is required to recognise in the characters Byron and Polidori, respectively, and in their tale, Polidori's story of their relationship.

In the tale itself, an unsuspecting Aubrey travels through Europe with Ruthven until he is finally made aware of his companion's malicious nature. Parting company with Ruthven, Aubrey first betrays his companion's evil intentions to the family of a prospective female victim before fleeing to Greece. It is in Greece that Aubrey meets the elf-like Ianthe, who, true to folk tradition, tells Aubrey of the existence of vampires (in which she wholly believes). Aubrey comes to see similarities between his former travel companion and the demonic souls of Ianthe's tales, but remains sceptical about such improbable connections. That is, until the day when poor Ianthe is killed by a vampire, and Ruthven follows close behind. Aubrey collapses. When Ruthven himself nurses him back to health, Aubrey again doubts his fears; and soon thereafter, when Ruthven dies of a gun-shot wound, Aubrey dismisses his suspicions and returns to London. This, of course, only after he ponders what might have happened to his friend's body, which has mysteriously disappeared.

In London, Aubrey returns to Society with his sister, who is courted by a mysterious stranger. The stranger, of course, proves to be Ruthven, who had solicited a solemn oath on his death-bed that Aubrey would tell no one of his death. Bound by his oath, Aubrey again falls ill, until finally he breaks his oath. He is dismissed as insane. Ruthven completes his revenge by effecting the fall of the house of Aubrey. Thus the modern vampire was born. In its birth are many of the themes we have since come to associate with the vampire: aristocratic background, hypnotic power over women, drinking of blood, eternal life, sociopathic destructiveness. The book was published in 1819, a year after Mary Shelley's *Frankenstein* and Blundell's first human transfusion. Initially appearing under Byron's name, "The Vampyre" became a highly influential success.[95]

Another tale in this genre – Edgar Allan Poe's *The Oval Portrait* – helps illuminate the similarities and differences between Frankenstein's monster and Polidori's vampire, and at the same time sets up the transformation from the vampiric to the scientific movement of blood between bodies. In it, an artist, fixated on painting his wife's image, does not notice that the woman's health is depleted in direct proportion to the progress he makes on the portrait. In Twitchell's words, "just as the painter finishes his work, he exclaims, 'This is indeed *Life* itself!' Enraptured, he turns from the painting to his wife, and, irony of ironies, she is dead."[96] The painting itself acts as a kind of creative force, draining vitality from its subject and thereby attaining life. Frankenstein's monster, also the object of art, comes to life through the combined vital forces of Victor and nature. And the vampire?

To cite Twitchell again, "vampires are not always foamy-mouthed fiends with blood dripping from extended incisors, but rather can be participants in some ghastly process of energy transfer in which one partner gains vitality at the expense of another."[97] The vampire draws vital energy, in the form of blood, from its subject, to recreate its own life. The vampire, the perverted personification of Romantic creativity, is its own creation. In other words, Frankenstein's monster was re-animated by an instrumentally guided electricity, whereas the vampire was re-animated more directly by another kind of vital substance: blood.

In the Romantic tales of Shelley and Polidori, as in the investigations of physiologically inclined medical men, blood and electricity are vital forces. Moreover, for both groups, blood and electricity are not creat*ed*, but creat*ive* – they are pre-existing vital forces that are harnessed by those who have learned their secrets. Such would also be the case for transfused blood.

Life's Blood

As did the medical unveilers who raised him, Blundell used apparent death and re-animation to create a place for himself at the death-bed. This place, however, took on a more distinctly material form for Blundell than it did for his teachers. For, from his own formulations, it is evident that Blundell thought of transfusion as a procedure capable of manipulating apparent death and directing it towards life. He explicitly compared its functions to resuscitation after submersion, and lamented the fate of those who did not receive its revitalising benefits before apparent death became real and irreversible.[98]

To appreciate the meanings transfusion is likely to have held for Blundell, let us look first at the recipients of transfusion in the 1820s. Primarily, these were women suffering and near death from uterine haemorrhage. At a time when man-midwives were still attempting to consolidate their power over the birthing process, Blundell offered another technical procedure – until now ignored by historians – that legitimated, even necessitated, a male practitioner's place in the birthing chamber. The transfusion-proficient accoucheur presided over the rebirth of the birthing mother. Descriptions of transfusion recipients, which consistently tell of their "death-like appearance," support this interpretation of transfusion as re-animation of the apparently dead.[99] Witness Blundell's Romantic description of the state of his transfused patients:

After floodings immediately, women sometimes die in a moment, but more frequently in a gradual manner; and over the victim death shakes his dart, and to you she stretches out her helpless hands for that assistance, which you cannot give, *unless by transfusion*.

I have seen a woman dying for two or three hours together, convinced in my own mind that no known remedy could save her; the sight of these moving cases first led me to transfusion ... The fatal termination is principally foreshown by a certain ghastliness of the countenance.[100]

One must not, however, wait *too* long to transfuse, or the woman will move from corpse-like to actual corpse – and will then be beyond blood's saving power.[101]

Compare this image of the woman in need of transfusion with Polidori's description of the murdered Ianthe in "The Vampyre:" "There was no colour upon her cheek, not even upon her lip; yet there was a stillness about her face that seemed almost as attaching as the life itself that once dwelt there." The cause of her unfortunate state is determined by the "marks of teeth having opened the vein" of her neck – placed there, we are told, by a "vampyre."[102] The vampiric Lord Ruthven is himself described as being of "deadly hue."[103] The analogies with blood transfusion are striking. A woman, corpse-like from loss of blood, lies near death. Now, however, she may yet be saved if the blood of a strong and healthy man is transfused *into* her. Moreover, this man might, in consequence of venesection, also grow pale and even be made to swoon: such is the nature of energy exchange by blood.

Beyond its application to apparent corpses, there is yet another place at which transfusion intersects with energy-exchanging re-animation. The striking scenes of women re-animated by transfused blood read as if they came from Shelley's pen – or Galvani's experimental accounts. Like the assembled pieces of diverse corpses or the dissected muscles of ambiguous frogs, these pale and transfused women suddenly jump to life, as if "reanimated by an electric spark."[104] In a culture attuned to the marvels of resuscitation and electrical stimulation, such reaction would at least have drawn medical attention, even convincing some of the re-animating potential of blood.

Turning now to the blood itself: what part did vitalistic notions of the blood play in early transfusion? Blundell's writings suggest that it was precisely his vital-materialist conception of blood that allowed him to consider transfusion as an effective therapeutic procedure. The very opening of his introductory physiology lecture of 1825 clearly set forth his views on vital principles:

When, again, directing our attention to the natural objects with which the globe abounds, we come to examine them with a little care, we find that a part of them, small in bulk though not in number, are in possession of powers of generation, and of taking up within themselves substances which are afterwards assimilated to their own nature; while others are destitute of these powers, and destitute also of that organisation and vital energy on which these powers depend.[105]

As we have seen, Blundell believed that physiological experimentation alone provides insight into the workings of these natural substances and allows us to manipulate them.

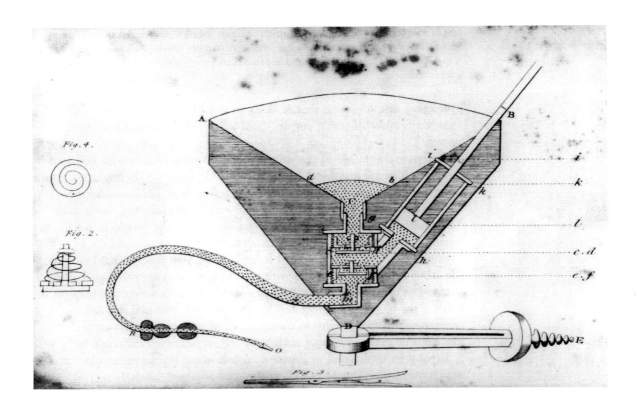

Figure 4. Blundell's 1824
Impellor illustrated in a
cut-away sketch that
reveals the maze through
which the blood was
moved.

Blundell's vitalistic conception of blood itself is evident in the way he
practised, and justified, transfusion – specifically, in the quantity of blood
he used, and the concerns he expressed about the instruments with which
he intended to move it between bodies. Concerning the amount of blood
used, *The Lancet* reported a case in which Blundell supplied only four
ounces, and afterwards admitted that some would question whether so little
blood "really saved the patient. The Doctor, however, (and he has seen a
great deal of haemorrhage) is decidedly of the opinion, that this timely
supply of vital fluid turned the scale in the patient's favour, and rescued her
from death."[106] Indeed, it was precisely the small amount of blood
transfused that Blundell's critics, assembled for a debate in 1825 at the
Medical Society of London, questioned as "not sufficient to explain the
improvement of the patient."[107] Blundell persevered in his commitment to
relatively small amounts of blood, which he thought sufficient to sustain
life.[108] Relatedly, Blundell also believed that the blood had a nutritive role
in the body, and that transfused blood sustained the system accordingly.
His vitalism, as I suggested earlier, was no longer the kind of active vitalism
espoused by Hunter, but the more materialistic variety that fitted into the
globular conceptions of his contemporaries.

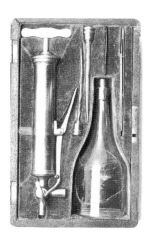

Figure 5. Syringe-based apparatus made in accordance with Blundell's specifications by Savigny, from the Wellcome collections at the Science Museum (A 43853).

Further evidence of Blundell's vitalistic perception of blood is suggested by his conception of the instruments with which he transfused it. Unlike the seventeenth-century transfusers, Blundell used blood from *human* donors. Animals might be subjected to arterial bleeding into quills or lengths of intestines connected to the veins of human recipients; however, as Blundell himself noted, "there are few perhaps but would object to the opening of an artery."[109] Consequently, he devised various instruments intended to replace the normal, artery-to-vein circulation. His first concern in devising these glass-and-brass instruments was whether "the blood would remain fit for the animal functions after its passage through the instrument."[110] Would the inanimate materials of instruments, he wondered, somehow destroy the very living qualities that gave blood its particular revitalising power? Each of his three transfusion apparatuses – the syringe, the "Impellor," and the Gravitator – he devised precisely to preserve the blood in its artificial movement from donating to receiving vein. The Impellor, introduced in 1824, relied on a receiving cup into which a maze of passages had been added, so as to preserve the motion of the blood as it was impelled by syringe through the cup (*see* Figure 4).

That Blundell's primary concern in constructing these elaborate pieces of apparatus was for preserving the blood's fitness in transfusion is evident in his stark admission that, "should it be found hereafter, by numerous pointed, and therefore decisive experiments and observations, that human blood may lie out of the vessels in the cup for several seconds, without becoming thereby unfit for the vital purposes … transfusion may be accomplished, by the syringe alone … on account of its greater simplicity."[111] Impellors and Gravitators, constructed in order to preserve the blood's fitness, would become superfluous (*see* Figure 5). Accordingly, it is clear that Blundell's was no simple quantitative belief in a direct replacement of haemorrhaged blood, but instead a more qualitative understanding of blood as life.

To complete my contextualising argument for the reintroduction of transfusion to British medical practice, I need to make a further, instrumental link. For, it could be argued, a great difference exists between Victor Frankenstein's rational manipulations of electrical nature and the vampire's rather folkloric sucking of blood. Where precisely does transfusion fit? Blundell's transfusion effectively shifts the movement of blood between bodies from the literary-sensuous to the clinical bedside. In other words, much like Victor Frankenstein, James Blundell has created instruments capable of directing vital forces towards chosen, re-animating ends. Let us recall again the few details of Frankenstein's creative moment with which Mary Shelley provides us: "I collected the instruments of life around me, that I might infuse a spark into the lifeless thing that lay at my feet."[112] Such could easily be a passage from one of Blundell's case histories of transfusion.

Indeed, the portrayal Blundell himself provided of transfusion by Gravitator makes my connecting case to Frankenstein clearer (*see* Figure 2). The 1828 Gravitator model dispensed entirely with the syringe, relying instead on a tall tube and – as the name implies – the force of gravity, to move the blood at a "proper" rate into the body. Pictured in the accompanying image are donor, receiver and instrument (including stream of blood). Like the Romantic genius–artist, Blundell, the Creator, is absent from the scene. He was its channel and now, what remains is the object of art – the transfusion scene – that he facilitated. Blundell *is* Victor; transfusion is Frankenstein's monster; both art-objects arise from proper understanding and instrumental channelling of nature's vital forces. One might even argue that James Blundell's instrumental interventions completed the vampire's movement from folk to Romantic figure. And, like Victor, Blundell ultimately suffered removal from society as a consequence of his hubris.

Does this mean that I read Blundell's medical innovation as a kind of Gothic tale-in-action? Not entirely. Comparison with the other famous gothic figure, the vampire, illustrates this qualification. Kininger's 1795 painting, "The Dream of Eleanor," is one in a genre of death-bed images that began with Henry Fuseli's famous "The Nightmare" (1781) and would be appropriated by nineteenth-century vampire enthusiasts (*see* Figure 6).[113] I have selected this particular permutation of Fuseli's image because "death," true to Blundell's descriptions, holds his "dart" above the woman (and her throat at that!). The similarities between Kininger's and Blundell's images do not end there. For, in both, the bed – presumably, the woman's bed – is the stage upon which the drama unfolds. The woman lying on the bed is the recipient of the drama's action; the male figure looming above her, the agent of that action. At this point, however, the images diverge. For in Kininger's piece, the woman's pose is one of sexual exhaustion. This posture contrasts strikingly with Blundell's transfusion recipient, who lies, passive, chaste and near death, on the bed. Blundell's transfusion recipient is perched on the edge of the Victorian age: the worthy mother in her bed-chamber, rather than the saucy victim of the vampire. Moreover, Kininger's agent is the cause of his victim's exhaustion, whereas Blundell's agent is the heroic restorer of energy otherwise lost. In short, the contrasting male figures embody the power of evil and of good.

The means by which transfuser and vampire move blood is also strikingly contrasted. We have seen an instrumental parallel between the vital channelling conducted by Blundell and Frankenstein. In comparison with vampires, however, we witness another difference of blood transfusion. For, connecting man and woman is no lusty blood-kiss or threatening dart, but a scientifically designed instrument. Rather like Laennec's device for auscultation (*see* Figure 7), Blundell's Gravitator provided an acceptable social distance between donor and recipient of blood, moving through

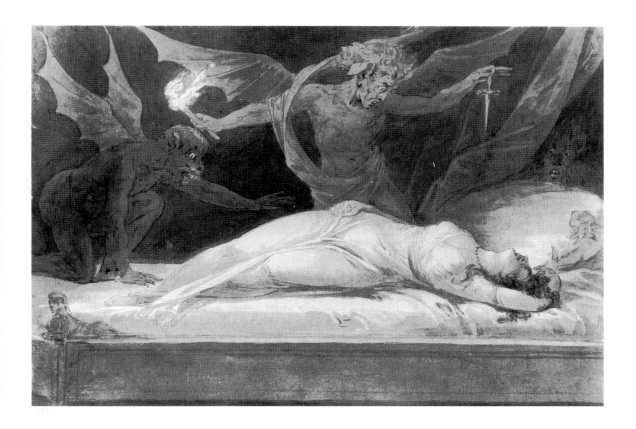

Figure 6. G. Kininger,
The Dream of Eleanor,
c. *1795.*

rationally designed and arranged instruments, and away from direct neck-biting.

In a sense, then, Blundell's innovation of transfusion relies on a re-animating conception of blood similar to the one that guides Polidori's vampire. At the same time, it asserts an alternative scenario – a clearly heroic place for the life-giving movement of blood between bodies. For Blundell, who was formed by the very London physicians who were busily creating a heroic professional image, gave transfusion a decidedly Romantic presentation. More than this, it is likely that the same re-animating sciences that encouraged elite medical practitioners at once to aspire to Promethean power over the line between life and death and to devise Romantic self-narratives, also provided the context in which blood transfusion made sense. Blundell's transfusion is a Romantic re-animation of the apparently dead. Cultural medical image fed substantive medical manifestation – rather like Odysseus feeding blood to the shades of Hades. Still, the Gothic remains, embodied in the ambiguous potential of an emergent biotechnology.

In this spirit, I would like to suggest a plausible "after" sketch of Blundell's sombre transfusion scene. The hero-husband would now be

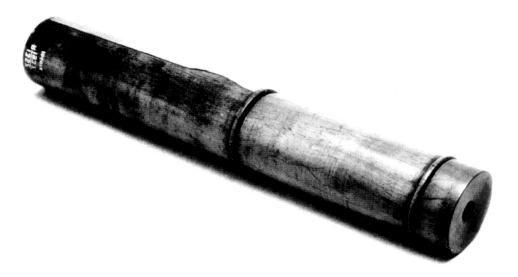

Figure 7. Laennec's stethoscope (c. 1820) provided an instrumentally-safe distance between doctor and patient. From the Wellcome collections at the Science Museum (A 106078).

seated, his head, perhaps, in his hands, as he attempts to restore his lost energy. The woman would certainly be wide-eyed and flushed. She might even be sitting upright as she exclaims to awe-struck medical witnesses: "By Jasus! I feel as strong as a bull!"[114]

Notes

This paper was made possible by the generous support of the Science Museum and the Wellcome Trust. Its arguments were strengthened by the suggestions of stimulating audiences at Cambridge University, the University of Manchester, Johns Hopkins University and the 1997 meeting of the AAHM. In particular I would like to thank Luke Davidson and Klif Fuller for sharing their expertise of life's darker corners, and Natsu Hattori for general inspiration and specific suggestions alike.

1. James Blundell, "Lectures on the Theory and Practice of Midwifery," *The Lancet* 1 (1827–28): 580. The lectures appear throughout the volume.
2. The French term was Blundell's choice, as opposed to the traditional "man-midwife".
3. See Kim Pelis, "Blood Clots: The 19th Century British Debate over the Substance and Means of Transfusion," *Annals of Science* 54 (1997): 331–60.
4. James Blundell, "Experiments on the Transfusion of Blood by the Syringe," *Medico-Chirurgical Transactions* 9 (1818): 56–92.
5. See A. D. Farr, "The First Human Blood Transfusion," *Medical History* 24 (1980): 143–62, 143, with expansion and corrections by A. Rupert Hall and Marie Boas Hall, "The First Human Blood Transfusion: Priority Disputes," *Medical History* 24 (1980): 461–65; Charles Waller, "Uterine Haemorrhage and Transfusion," *The Lancet* 10 (1826): 58–62; Simon Schaffer, "The Body of Natural Philosophers in Restoration England," in *Knowledge Incarnate: The Physical Presentation of Intellectual Selves*, ed. Christopher Lawrence and Steven Shapin (Chicago, 1998): 51–82.
6. In his introductory chapter, Chris Baldick (*In Frankenstein's Shadow* [Oxford, 1987]) provides an excellent introduction to the issues concerning post-revolutionary Europe.
7. For introductory purposes, I use the problematic term "Romantic" quite generally, allowing it to contain numerous periods and national styles. For a recent review of the "problematic" aspects of the term in the history of science, see Trevor H. Levere, "Romanticism, Natural Philosophy and the Science: A Review and Bibliographic Essay," *Perspectives on Science* 4 (1996): 463–88. I shall qualify the term further below.

8. Simon Schaffer, "Genius in Romantic Natural Philosophy," in *Romanticism and the Sciences*, ed. Andrew Cunningham and Nicholas Jardine (Cambridge, 1990), pp. 82–98; Ludmilla Jordanova, "Melancholy Reflection: Constructing an Identity for Unveilers of Nature," in *Frankenstein, Creation and Monstrosity*, ed. Stephen Bann (London, 1994), pp. 60–76.

9. Luke Davidson, "Chapter 1", unpublished manuscript from his dissertation on the Royal Humane Society and apparent death; David Knight, "Romanticism and the Sciences," in Cunningham and Jardine, eds. (n. 8 above), pp. 13–24; Martin Pernick, "Back from the Grave: Recurring Controversies over Defining and Diagnosing Death in History," in *Death: Beyond Whole–Brain Criteria*, ed. Richard M. Zaner (Dordrecht and Boston, 1988), pp. 17–74.

10. Dorothy Porter and Roy Porter, *Patient's Progress: Doctors and Doctoring in 18th Century England* (Cambridge, 1989), p. 171.

11. While the vampire enjoyed a long and healthy life in Eastern European folk tradition, it is seen to have been introduced to "high" culture with John Polidori's 1819 story, "The Vampyre." See Christopher Frayling, *Vampyres: Lord Byron to Count Dracula* (London, 1991); James B. Twitchell, *The Living Dead: A Study of the Vampire in Romantic Literature* (Durham, NC, 1981). The recent academic conference, "Frankenfest," testifies to the interest held by historians of science in Mary Shelley's classic tale. See also Tim Marshall, *Murdering to Dissect: Grave-Robbing, Frankenstein and the Anatomy Literature* (Manchester, 1995); Baldick (n. 6 above).

12. For a review of English themes, see Marilyn Butler, "Romanticism in England," in *Romanticism in National Context*, ed. Roy Porter and Mikulas Teich (Cambridge, 1988), pp. 37–67. On Romanticism and science, Butler's "Introduction" to Mary Shelley's *Frankenstein, or the Modern Prometheus* [1818 text] (Oxford, 1993); and Jordanova (n. 8 above) as well as her essay review, "Romantic Science? Michelet, Morals, and Nature," *British Journal for the History of Science* 13 (1980): 44–50.

13. I will be dealing with the obstetrical dimensions of transfusion only superficially in this paper. A fuller treatment will be given to these questions in my forthcoming book on British transfusion.

14. I have filled this out with the words of various contributors to *The Lancet*, the medical journal that staunchly supported transfusion (this during its first decade of publication).

15. To name but a few studies of this nexus of ideas as they relate to science: Marcello Pera, *The Ambiguous Frog: The Galvani–Volta Controversy on Animal Electricity* (Princeton, 1992); Desmond King-Hele, *Erasmus Darwin and the Romantic Poets* (London, 1986); Luke Davidson, "Pursuing a Cultural History of Death: The Royal Humane Society and Apparent Death, 1774–1800," unpublished manuscript, presented December 1996, Wellcome Institute Research in Progress Seminar; Charlotte Sleigh, *Life, Death and Galvanism*, unpublished manuscript, presented October 1996, Wellcome Research in Progress Seminar; Ruth Richardson, *Death, Dissection and the Destitute* (London, 1987).

16. The stated reasons for Blundell's unexpected retirement are discussed in a series of letters to *The Lancet*. Apparently, the treasurer of Guy's Hospital named one Samuel Ashwell co-chair with Blundell – much to Blundell's chagrin and stated surprise. It would seem that political alliances and relations with *The Lancet* itself were also factors in Blundell's departure. See "Dr. Blundell's Reasons for his Retirement from the Medical School of Guy's Hospital," *The Lancet* 1 (1834–35): 28–32. The discussion continues with a reply from his adversary, Samuel Ashwell, pp. 78–79; Blundell's "Second Letter to his Medical Friends," pp. 207–12; Ashwell, again, pp. 259–61; and Blundell's "Third Letter," pp. 418–25.

17. I have taken basic biographical details from the following sources: Charles Waller, "On Transfusion of Blood: Its History, and Application in cases of Severe Haemorrhage," *Transactions of the Obstetrical Society of London* 1 (1859): 61–72; "Obituary: James Blundell," *British Medical Journal* 1 (1878): 351–52; "Obituary: James Blundell," *The Lancet* 1 (1878): 255–56; J. H. Young, "James Blundell (1790–1878): Experimental Physiologist and Obstetrician," *Medical History* 8 (1964): 159–69; B. A. Myhre, "James Blundell – Pioneer Transfusionist," *Transfusion* 35 (1995): 74–78.

18. "Obituary," *The Lancet* 1 (1878): 255.

19. *Dictionary of National Biography* (London, 1890), p. 441, v. 23. This conception is confirmed in "Review, Blundell, *The Principles and Practice of Obstetricy,* by Thomas Castle," *The Edinburgh Medical and Surgical Journal* 42 (1834): 138–55, 140.

20. An amusing example of this particular gift is cited in "One Hundred Years Ago: The Teaching of Midwifery in London in 1814: Haighton and Blundell," *British Medical Journal* 2 (1914): 21–23. This article also draws attention to Blundell's success, calling it "phenomenal": "for years he had the largest class on midwifery in London" (p. 21).

21. If nothing else, the fictional voice allows the post-modern historian to add a rare word to her text.

22. "Comments on the Speeches at the Anniversary Dinner of St. Thomas's and Guy's Hospitals," *The Lancet* 1 (1823–24): 422.

23. "Dr. Blundell's Introductory Physiology Lecture," *The Lancet* 9 (1825–26): 118. Vathek is a character from William Beckford's 1786 story, *Vathek: An Arabian Tale*. Apparently, the story influenced the imagination of Byron as well as Blundell.

24. James Blundell, "Some Remarks on the Operation of Transfusion," in *Researches Physiological and Pathological: Instituted Principally with a View to the Improvement of Medical and Surgical Practice* (London, 1824), p. 69.

25. On "passive vitality," see "Dr. Blundell's Introductory Physiology Lecture" (n. 23 above), p. 114.

26. Blundell (n. 24 above), p. 123.

27. I have compiled this fictional case from a number of accounts given in *The Lancet* during the 1820s and early 30s. See, for example, 9 (1825–26): 11, 295; 10 (1826): 280; 1 (1828–29): 431; 1 (1834): 156–57.

28. "Transfusion of Blood in Uterine Haemorrhage," *The Lancet* 1(1834–35): 157.

29. "Case of Uterine Haemorrhage, in which the Operation of Transfusion was Successfully Performed, by Charles Waller, M.D.," *The Lancet* 1 (1833–34): 522.

30. "Successful Case of Transfusion. by J. Howell, esq., Bridge Street, Southwark," *The Lancet* 1 (1827–28): 698.

31. James Blundell, "Observations on Transfusion of Blood, with a Description of his Gravitator," *The Lancet* 2 (1828–29): 321–24.

32. Blundell (n. 4 above), pp. 56–57.

33. "Transfusion of Blood" (n. 28 above), p. 156.

34. Ibid., p. 157.

35. Jos. Ralph, "Another Successful Case of Transfusion," *The Lancet* 10 (1826): 280.

36. Charles Waller, *Elements of Practical Midwifery, or, Companion to the Lying-In Room* (London, 1829), pp. 89, 91.

37. Waller (n. 5 above), p. 60. It is quite possible that the friendly support Blundell enjoyed from Wakley and *The Lancet* played a role in his ultimate retirement from Guy's in 1834. Guy's and St Thomas's had been the focus of consistent attack – for nepotism, inadequacy, and a kind of medical despotism – by Wakley's journal, with the hospitals' treasurer coming under particular attack. It was this same treasurer who precipitated Blundell's actions. On Wakley, see Richardson (n. 15 above), pp. 42–50; S. Squire Sprigge, *The Life and Times of Thomas Wakley*, facsimile of the 1899 edition (Huntington, NY, 1974).

38. In his classic study *The Vampire* (London, 1995), originally published in 1928, Montague Summers examines the connections between this fear and vampire legends in some detail. More recently, historians and anthropologists have attended to funeral rituals of various times and cultures. Richardson gives wonderful descriptive analyses of laying out corpses in *Death, Dissection and the Destitute* (n. 15 above). For an anthropological perspective, see Nigel Barley, *Dancing on the Grave* (London, 1995).

39. On French "vitalistic materialism," see Owsei Temkin, "The Philosophical Background of Magendie's Physiology," and "Materialism in French and German Physiology of the Early 19th Century," *Bulletin of the History of Medicine* 20 (1946): 10–35 and 322–27, respectively.

40. Knight (n. 9 above), pp. 19–21; Davidson, *Chapter 1* (n. 9 above).

41. Davidson (n. 15 above), pp. 3–4.

42. The Humane Society's techniques are reviewed in L. H. Hawkins, "The History of Resuscitation," *British Journal of Hospital Medicine* 4 (1970): 495–500.

43. Davidson (n. 15 above), pp. 9–10.

44. Ibid., pp. 10–11.

45. Pera (n. 15 above), pp. 3–18.

46. Sleigh (n. 15 above).

47. Davidson (n. 15 above), p. 11.

48. Erwin Ackerknecht, *Medicine at the Paris Hospital, 1794–1848* (Baltimore, 1967); Toby Gelfand, *Professionalizing Modern Medicine: Paris Surgeons and Institutions in the 18th Century* (Westport, Conn., 1980).

49. Knight (n. 9 above), pp. 19–20.

50. Christopher Lawrence, "The Nervous System and Society in the Scottish Enlightenment," in *Natural Order: Historical Studies of Scientific Culture*, ed. Barry Barnes and Steven Shapin (Beverly Hills and London, 1979), pp. 19–40, discusses in detail the Edinburgh conception of the body and the ways it fitted into Scottish notions of society and civility. His summary of Cullen's work is on p. 26. On the rise of vitalism in the mid-eighteenth century, see Theodore M. Brown, "From Mechanism to Vitalism in 18th-Century English Physiology," *Journal of the History of Biology* 7 (1974): 217–58. On its abrupt German, and more gradual French, decline after the 1830s, see Everett Mendelsohn, "Physical Models and Physiological Concepts: Explanation in 19th-Century Biology," *British Journal for the History of Science* 2 (1965): 201–19.

51. Almost every history of blood or transfusion opens with a paragraph, or even a chapter, on this persistent belief that "the blood is the life." Jean-Paul Roux has provided a broad-ranging and nuanced study of the meanings of blood in antiquity, in *Le sang: Mythes, symboles et réalités* (Paris, 1988). For a lighter introduction to the history of moving blood between bodies, see Kim Pelis, "Moving Blood," *Vox Sanguinis*, 73 (1997): 201–6.

52. Everett Mendelsohn, *Heat and Life* (Cambridge, Mass., 1964), p. 29; Schaffer (n. 8 above).

53. John Pickstone, "Globules and Coagula: Concepts of Tissue Formation in the Early Nineteenth Century," *Journal of the History of Medicine and the Allied Sciences* 28 (1973): 336–56, 339. A detailed, if reverent, critique of Hunter's vitalistic conception of blood is given in C. Turner Thackrah, *An Inquiry into the Nature and Properties of the Blood, as Existent in Health and Disease* (London, 1819). Lawrence (n. 50 above), p. 34, states explicitly that Hunter located the "living principle" in blood, as contrasted with the Edinburgh school's focus on the "nervous fluid."

54. Temkin, "Materialism" (n. 39 above).

55. Pickstone (n. 53 above), pp. 345–47. It should also be noted that Prevost and Dumas began to experiment on transfusion and defibrination of the blood in 1821.

56. Diana Manuel, "Marshall Hall (1790–1857): Vivisection and the Development of Experimental Physiology," in *Vivisection in Historical Perspective*, ed. Nicolaas A. Rupke (London, 1987), pp. 78–104.

57. Butler, "Introduction" (n. 12 above), pp. xviii–xxi.

58. Jordanova (n. 8 above), pp. 61–62. Schaffer connects similar qualities to his description of Romantic genius. Schaffer (n. 8 above), pp. 93–94.

59. Jordanova (n. 8 above), pp. 72–73. I would like to add an interesting twist to Jordanova's argument. She dismisses the possibility that Mary Shelley was thinking about surgeons as she conceived of her monster, because "surgery was active and manual, but not until the second half of the nineteenth century did it entail much entry into body cavities" (p. 66). This is certainly true on a general level. Blundell, however, was writing treatises on abdominal surgery and conducting animal experiments to show its potential in the 1810s – further substantiating his "frankensteinian" character!

60. I draw this analogy from Butler's arguments about Romanticism and the Gothic novel ("Romanticism in England" [n. 12 above], pp. 62–63) and Jordanova's accounts of medical self-image and Frankenstein's character (n. 8 above).

61. Levere (n. 7 above), p. 466; Jordanova (n. 8 above), p. 62; Knight (n. 9 above), pp. 19–20; Schaffer (n. 8 above), pp. 91–94; Cunningham and Jardine, "The Age of Reflection," in Cunningham and Jardine, eds. (n. 8 above), p. 6.

62. Davidson discusses the cultural consequences of this shift in "apparent death" extensively in the opening chapter of his dissertation, in progress.

63. "Creating a *culture* of medical and scientific power was one way of securing power itself." Jordanova (n. 8 above), p. 67.

64. Butler, "Romanticism in England" (n. 12 above), p. 37; Morse Peckham, *Romanticism and Ideology* (Hanover, NH, 1995), pp. 3–4; Knight (n. 9 above), p. 13.

65. Issues concerning national styles of Romanticism guide the essays in Porter and Teich (n. 12 above).

66. Knight (n. 9 above), p. 13.
67. In Randy Shilts' book and the movie based upon it – *And the Band Played On: Politics, People, and the AIDS Epidemic* (London, 1988) – the Centers for Disease Control's tireless AIDS campaigner, Dr Donald Francis, is given just such a Romantic description.
68. Butler, "Romanticism in England" (n. 12 above), pp. 56–60.
69. The classic study of this "orientalising" tendency and its history is Edward W. Said, *Orientalism* (New York, 1979).
70. King-Hele (n. 15 above), chap. 8.
71. Numerous dissertations of the Royal Medical Society, the elite student society in Edinburgh, treat galvanism and the resuscitation of the drowned. See, for example, W. B. Almon, "What are the properties of Galvanism?", pp. 1808–09, v. 61; Thomas Reive, "What is the best mode of recovering suspended animation?", pp. 1810–11, v. 65. Edinburgh University, *Special Collections; Royal Medical Society Index to Dissertations F/N96935/1.*
72. On Edinburgh medical education in this period, see Lisa Rosner, *Medical Education in the Age of Improvement: Edinburgh Students and Apprentices, 1760–1826* (Edinburgh, 1991); L. S. Jacyna, *Philosophic Whigs: Medicine, Science and Citizenship in Edinburgh, 1789–1848* (London, 1994); Christopher Lawrence, "The Edinburgh Medical School and the End of the 'Old Thing,' 1790–1830," in *History Of Universities* (Oxford, 1988), vol. 3, pp. 259–86.
73. Joannes Davies, "De Mortu Varae Indiciis," (MD diss. Edinburgh University, 1813).
74. Jacobus Blundell, "De Sensu quo Melos Sentitur," (MD diss. Edinburgh University, 1813). Blundell dedicates his dissertation to Haighton.
75. Of course, at the time, dissection was particularly stigmatised by the general use of the bodies of executed criminals for medical study. See Richardson (n. 15 above); Marshall (n. 11 above).
76. James Moores Ball, *The Body Snatchers* (New York, 1989).
77. Richardson (n. 15 above) and Marshall (n. 11 above) both discuss the class dimensions of dissections and the Anatomy Act. It is apparent that at least some of the women transfused by Blundell were of the lower classes. I have not examined the gender and class dimensions of the transfusion story systematically, though I would suspect that they parallel that of forceps.
78. "Dr. Blundell's Introductory Physiology Lecture" (n. 23 above), pp. 115–16.
79. Malcolm Jack, ed., *Vathek and Other Stories: A William Beckford Reader* (London, 1995), pp. 27–121.
80. Butler, "Introduction" (n. 12 above), pp. xxvi–xxvii.
81. "Comments on the Speeches" (n. 22 above).
82. The famous image of a similarly-clad Byron springs to mind. *The Lancet* 7 (1825): 146–47. Having described Blundell, *The Lancet* continued: "We are sorry to say many were present who had *no characters.*"
83. Thomas Castle, *The Principles and Practice of Obstetricy, as at Present Taught by James Blundell* (London, 1834), pp. 419, 420.
84. Marriage, at least. Blundell was a life-long bachelor.
85. By "conceived," I refer to their birth into "polite literary society." The vampire myth in particular had long existed in folk tales.
86. Mary Shelley herself appears to have set off the controversy in her introduction to the 1831 edition of *Frankenstein*, in which she essentially dismisses Polidori and his influence on her novel. In his study, *Vampyres: Lord Byron to Count Dracula*, Christopher Frayling attempts to restore creative credibility to Polidori's name. The episode is also discussed by Butler ("Introduction" [n 12 above]) and Twitchell (n. 11 above).
87. Franklin Bishop, *Polidori! A Life of Dr. John Polidori* (Kent, 1991).
88. I am referring to the first edition of *Frankenstein*, published in 1818. See Baldick (n. 6 above), chap. 1.
89. Shelley (n. 12 above), p. 24. The 1831 edition adds "galvanism."
90. Ibid., p. 34.
91. Ibid., pp. 36–37.
92. Ibid., p. 38.
93. Twitchell (n. 11 above), pp. 142–43.
94. John Polidori, "The Vampyre," reprinted with Shelley's *Frankenstein* (London, 1992), p. 236.

95. Frayling (n. 11 above) and Twitchell (n. 11 above) both discuss the literary influence of Polidori's creation.
96. Twitchell (n. 11 above), p. 166.
97. Ibid., p. 3.
98. See above quotations, cited in notes 1 and 24.
99. Ralph (n. 35 above), p. 280.
100. Blundell (n. 1 above), p. 614.
101. Blundell experimented with animals to determine how long one might wait to transfuse, and found that at "actual death" the animal was, indeed, too far gone to resuscitate. In 1826, an experiment was conducted by Mr Scott at Guy's Hospital on a man actually dead; no positive result was noted as a consequence of the transfusion. "Transfusion," *The Lancet* 10 (1826): 221. In one of history's wonderful turns, about a century later, cadavers were employed as blood *donors* in parts of Russia – death quickly killed off unfortunate blood-borne infections and staved off coagulation. The procedure never caught on broadly, though it is nicely documented in the uncut version of the 1941 Paul Rotha film, "Blood Transfusion."
102. Polidori, cited in Twitchell (n. 11 above), p. 110.
103. Ibid., p. 236.
104. "Transfusion of Blood" (n. 28 above).
105. "Dr. Blundell's Introductory Physiology Lecture" (n. 23 above), p. 111.
106. "Transfusion," *The Lancet* 8 (1825): 343.
107. "Medical Society of London," *The Lancet* 9 (1825–26): 134.
108. Blundell (n. 4 above), p. 75; Waller (n. 5 above), p. 58.
109. Blundell (n. 4 above), p. 64.
110. Blundell (n. 24 above), pp. 56–57.
111. Ibid., p. 127. The Wellcome collections, housed at the Science Museum, London (WC/SM), includes a Blundell syringe-based transfusion apparatus, inv. no. A 43853. *See* Figure 5.
112. Shelley (n. 12 above), p. 38.
113. Twitchell (n. 11 above) examines these images in connection with vampire representations in his first chapter. I am not arguing that Kininger was attempting to portray a vampire in this painting – though the slightly pointed incisors and bat-like wings of the male image might support this claim. Instead, with Twitchell, I appeal to it primarily because illustrators looking for visual representations of nineteenth-century vampire stories used it, with Fuseli, as a model. Of course, this coincidence of images raises suggestive questions for cultural history – questions which I must, unfortunately, leave aside for the purposes of this paper.
114. "Another Successful Case of Transfusion," *The Lancet* 9 (1825–26): 111–12, 112.

Klaus Vogel

The Transparent Man – some comments on the history of a symbol

The desire to peer into the interior of the human body is ancient, but the realisation of this dream has, typically, required the destruction of life. In Christian societies, this has been regarded as a sinful injury of the body that God gave to man, and across cultures and historical epochs such mutilation has been a taboo as strong as the urge for knowledge. An alternative means of acquiring knowledge of the interior of the human body is offered by the "Transparent Man," the transparent model that has been on display in the German Hygiene Museum in Dresden since 1930.[1] The model, whose German name "Gläserner Mensch" can be translated literally as the "glass human," is life-size and, under a transparent plastic skin, contains the light metal mould of a human skeleton, with artificial internal organs, coloured and accurately shaped and arranged, and the arterial, venous and lymphatic systems represented by finely rolled painted wire. The Transparent Man is not made of glass: "Gläsern" is simply a metaphor for its transparency. How did this model come to be envisaged; how was it brought into being; how is one to view it now?

For all its transparency, there is an ambivalence about the model: it can be seen in terms of both entertainment and enlightenment, in terms of cultural symbolism within diverse traditions, and even in terms of its commercial value. What role, one may ask, can the Transparent Man have in the context of modern health care? Its historical significance gives the model additional interest: it has associations with the history of the German Hygiene Museum and, more broadly, with nearly a century of Germany's past.[2]

The Open Body – Anatomy, Dissection and Abduction Twixt Repulsion and Delight[3]

Before examining the aesthetics and accuracy of portrayal, let us consider the layperson's impressions of modern anatomical dissection. I visited the study galleries of the Institute for Anatomy at the Medical Faculty of the Dresden Technical University. Three groups, each of about ten students, and each guided by a postgraduate, were operating on three bodies. My visit took place towards the beginning of the semester, so the dissection of the bodies had not yet progressed very far. Early fear that I would have to leave the room in haste proved unfounded. This was due largely to the carefully considered environment, the good lighting, excellent ventilation, and the preceding preparation of the bodies that still exuded a softly sweetish alcoholic scent. The quietly concentrated activity of the young students, together with the friendly voice of my guide, were calculated to subdue any sensation of unmitigated horror.

This sobriety of the modern anatomical preparation room, and the sensation of an unusual but not horrific activity, are in extreme contrast to anatomy as experienced by Hector Berlioz in the nineteenth century. He recounts his participation at a dissection: "The appearance of this human meat hall, of chopped-off body parts, of grimacing heads, of the bloody cesspit in which we were running around, the disgusting smell that emanated from all this, it filled me with such disgust that I could not help fleeing, jumped through the window of the Anatomy, and rushed off as if Death himself with all his followers were chasing me."[4]

There is a reverse side to horror: fascination. The anatomical demonstration room was as much a site of feelings of sensationalism as of research. The proximity of death without sorrow, the "high" of shock, the attraction of the sensational on the borderline of the bearable – all this might be experienced by the layperson both as horror and as titillation, although nowadays it is probably more readily communicated in blood-curdling measure through the modern mass media of cinema, TV and video.

How different the Transparent Man: glass-like and totally intact, whose smooth exterior contains well-ordered organs undisturbed by intermediate tissues, with intermittent illumination for some, but by no means all!

Excursion Into Anatomy: *Ancestors and Founders of Anatomy – Dürer, Leonardo da Vinci, Vesalius*

The Transparent Man can be understood as a twentieth-century attempt to express the human form artistically. Such endeavours have, of course, a great ancestry. Without possibly being comprehensive, it is worth reflecting on some of the artists of the sixteenth century who sought accuracy in addition to a new depth of expression. For them, creating a likeness of the human body presupposed knowledge of the human subject, but their approaches to an exact understanding of the human *corpus* differed.

Albrecht Dürer (1471–1528) stands for the observing and measuring eye: both in his artistic works and in his theoretical instructions he displayed a sensitivity to the exact mensuration of the human body.[5] Nonetheless, he kept away from the dissecting table, relying on ruler, compass, wire-frame surround and the precepts of proportion for his extremely accurate images of man's proportions. The precision of measurement replaced the mutilation of tissue. Accurate observation was not an end in itself for Dürer, but was intended to serve the portrayal of the diversity of human appearance in a new way: he sought to represent living and respiring bodies. In gauntness, age or illness, or in contentedness, dignity and pride, they all come to life in Dürer's work with an intensity that moves the observer even today.

An alternative path was taken by Dürer's contemporary, Leonardo da Vinci (1452–1519). Leonardo the artist, philosopher and engineer – and also anatomist – ventured to explore the unknown and the unimaginable. The portrayals of the human body that Leonardo found in existing teaching texts did not accord with his own anatomical observations. That, as much as his urge for exploration, may have urged him to perform his own dissections. The sketches made on these occasions are of impressive accuracy and match even today's critical demands. At the same time, one is struck by the liveliness of the portrayals in Leonardo's anatomical studies: the bodies are not schematised, they are not anonymous; they show individuality, even emotion. This shows, on the one hand, Leonardo's mastery, both as anatomist and as artist, and, on the other, his search for underlying human dynamics. As humanist, he was not so much in quest of the mechanical body functions: in his anthropology, questions of art and science, philosophy and religion, all carried equal weight. Leonardo's studies do not just delineate corporeal structures; they reveal, through their omission of intermediate layers, a direct view into the human body.[6]

Conventionally, the creation of modern anatomy has been ascribed to Andreas Vesalius (1514–64). Born in Flanders, in 1537 he was eventually appointed to the first Chair for Surgery and Anatomy in Padua. With his exact observations, Vesalius overthrew the classical teachings of Galen that had hitherto been regarded as near sacrosanct. He published his epoch-making work, *De humani corporis fabrica libri septem*, in 1543:[7] "muscle men" appear upright, in movement from picture to picture, against the background of an idealised Tuscan landscape. No longer "corpse on dissecting table," but aesthetic appeal, the head stretched towards heaven, whilst the musculature is supported upon the earth.

Rays and Words – Röntgen and Freud
At the turn of the twentieth century, two new fields opened up hitherto unattainable insights into the human body – entirely without scalpel, without dissection and without the necessity of death – and aroused enormous public interest: X-ray imaging and psychoanalysis.

Wilhelm Conrad Röntgen (1845–1923), a physicist working in Würzburg, Bavaria, had discovered that, in experiments with electric tubes, rays were released that were also capable of penetrating through solid materials. To distinguish them from other rays, Röntgen called them "X-rays," and in his first publication he stated that various materials showed varying degrees of permeability to the rays.[8] From the earliest experiments, human bodies were irradiated and the early X-ray pioneers often used themselves, particularly their own hands, for tests. Medical applications evolved in parallel with the development and establishment of the new technology, and even became the force driving the testing of and further research on, the physical phenomenon.

From today's perspective, the rapid dissemination of knowledge about the new technique in the widest of circles appears quite as astonishing as the phenomenon itself. Röntgen discovered the effect in November 1895; it was first published at the turn of the year 1895/96, and as early as January 13, 1896 Röntgen was able to show his experiments to the German Kaiser, Wilhelm II. Not just scientists were enthused by the novel experience of looking inside the body: the idea of the irradiated human quickly took root in caricatures and presentations in the popular press, theatre and elsewhere. Curiosity and fascination with the clear and entirely bloodless pictures and insights went hand in hand with a smirking voyeurism, which today finds its last dregs in so-called "X-ray spectacles" obtainable as joke items.[9]

At almost the same time as the discovery and triumphant progress of X-rays, psychoanalysis – a quite different approach, which would illuminate another aspect of the innermost part of man – was developed by an equally deep and courageous thinker. Sigmund Freud (1856–1939), whose career as a doctor and scientist in Vienna after his medical studies had not been particularly successful, was influenced by the work of Charcot, who achieved therapeutic successes with hypnosis at the Salpêtrière Hospital in Paris.[10] His experiences in Paris, his attentive observation of his patients and, not least, the reflection of his own subconscious experience, led Freud painfully, step by step, to formulate his psychoanalytical philosophy. One of the first milestones was his theory of the meaning of dreams, which was published in 1899.[11] Further epoch-making works, *Psychopathology of Everyday Life* and *Three Essays on Sexual Theory* soon followed, in 1901 and 1905. Neither the scalpel nor the microscope but, purely and simply, words, had become the instrument for opening up insights for which there had been no precedent in conventional therapy.

Whereas Röntgen's discovery has its continuation in the highest development of modern image-producing processes, Freud's theory exerted its effects far into the fields of literature and art. The challenge of seeing into man, with its appeals to enlightenment and credulity that have always been ambiguous, has attracted an interest that lies beyond the narrow confines of science.

The Prehistory: A New Type of Exhibition – Hygiene Exhibitions

Millions of people have viewed and admired the Transparent Man in museums and exhibitions. To understand the phenomenon of this continuing interest, one has to consider the context in which this new art form was first presented. The forum for presentation of these transparent figures was a new type of exhibition: the social and hygiene (healthy living) exhibitions, and museums. At the end of the nineteenth century, the museum, originally created as a showplace of rarities for delectation of the nobility, and later as a forum for bourgeois devotion and strengthened self-assurance, gained a wholly new quality: as medium and as instrument of education. Contemporary with the development of social legislation in Germany, this new type of exhibition found its place in education and improvement, and thus was able to compete with the more far-reaching aspirations for emancipation by a working-class movement that was growing ever stronger.[12]

These enterprises were supported by the state, but also by private companies that wished to promote the spread of knowledge of hygiene and an appreciation of safety at work among the workers. Rapid industrialisation prompted rapid urban growth that was accompanied by inadequate sanitation. Concern for the preservation of a healthy working class, seen as vital to good productivity, prompted a multitude of hygienic endeavours. Under the guidance of Max Pettenkofer, a Chair in Hygiene was established by Munich University in 1865. Such men as Pettenkofer, Rudolf Virchow and Robert Koch not only had responsibility for the outcome of new research, they demanded prophylactic and educational steps towards the promotion of good health.

Early experience in building great international exhibitions was gained in the second half of the nineteenth century in France and in England.[13] Exhibitions gained impetus from trade and industry exhibitions that culminated in the well-known world exhibitions. The world exhibition of 1867, in Paris, provided an opportunity for more than 600 enterprises to exhibit in a section for social services, where aspects of medical care and hygiene were given prominence. Eventually, in 1882, Berlin hosted a first-rate hygiene exhibition that was sponsored by the German Association for Public Health Care.

These exhibitions all showed a wide range of model installations and equipment, and the results of research into medicine and hygiene were also exhibited in an easy-to-understand manner. Thus, in the 1883 German General Exhibition for Hygiene and Safety, next to Robert Koch's bacteriological researches were exhibited new designs for working-class housing, models of modern public baths, and equipment for the mechanical production of ice and Nestlé's substitute for human milk.[14] This trio of health education, industrial exhibition and scientific forum was also to be encountered in other hygiene exhibitions and museums.

Out of the Berlin exhibition, which had enjoyed great success with 900,000 visitors, arose the first Berlin Hygiene Museum. There were other state initiatives, and a corporate initiative worthy of mention: the AEG Hygiene Museum, dedicated to maintenance of the fitness of employees for work. Here, dramatic illustrations with models and life-like wax reproductions served to demonstrate the consequences of works injuries, poor nutrition or sexual diseases. An exhibition of prostheses was opened after the First World War, in response to the urgent requirements of the time.[15]

These public health and hygiene exhibitions were, typically, supported by the most modern technology of museum exhibition and teaching, incorporating demonstrations using working machines, slide shows and instructive films. Outside the major urban centres, the wider public were able to visit touring exhibitions. Through these museums and exhibits, the individual was guided towards a "sensible" lifestyle.

Following the formation of the Berlin Hygiene Museum, social and health concerns and aspirations current within the Kingdom of Saxony and its capital, Dresden (about 100 miles south of Berlin), led to a discussion of the merits of a local museum of hygiene. In 1883, the Dresden Association for the Protection of Nature and for Health Care addressed a "Petition for the Institution of a Hygiene Museum" to the country's Parliament.[16] While well received, the petition, for the moment, failed.

This Dresden vision was, nonetheless, ultimately realised, thanks to an extraordinary entrepreneurial personality: Karl August Lingner (1861–1916), inventor and marketing genius of the mouthwash "Odol."[17] He had earned a fortune based on new scientific insight into infections and the importance of oral hygiene, and on the inspired promotion of a brand name. His entrepreneurial ambitions were matched by a commitment to enlightenment and to social concerns, demonstrated by a multiplicity of charitable foundations. Lingner knew how to utilise modern means for large-scale exhibitions. Within the context of the great Dresden exhibition of 1903, "The German Cities," he organised a special show with the title *Popular Illnesses and the Means for Combating Them*. More than 200,000 visitors saw this exhibition, on which Lingner commented:

This special exhibition was founded on the awareness that echoes, like a cry for help, through all social-political utterances, the conviction that the centre of gravity of all social hygienic activities lies in the hygiene education of the population ...[18]

Lingner laid out the exhibition along the lines of a textbook. The exhibition hall was structured as three chapters: *Origin*, *Spread*, and *Fight Against Population Diseases*. He laid greatest stress on accessible displays, and the material for instruction and exhibition had been specially commissioned for the exhibition. Amongst others, there were bacterial cultures, viewable through microscopes, much enlarged models of bacteria, alcohol-preserved medical exhibits and wax models of the manifestations of various diseases, complemented by well-designed explanatory tables and statistics.

The success of this 1903 exhibition gave impetus to a much more significant project. On May 6, 1911, the First International Hygiene Exhibition opened in Dresden, under the aegis of the City of Dresden, the Kingdom of Saxony, and the German State. With 30 participating nations, around 100 specially erected exhibition buildings, and more than 5 million visitors, the enterprise could truly claim the status of an international exhibition. It was a milestone not just on account of its size, but because of its structure, which was in the vanguard of pedagogical practice and novelty of exhibits.

The Models of Spalteholz at the 1911 Hygiene Exhibition

The transparent organs on the *Der Mensch* (*Man*) stand were unprecedented, and proved a magnet for visitors. In 1906, the Leipzig medical practitioner

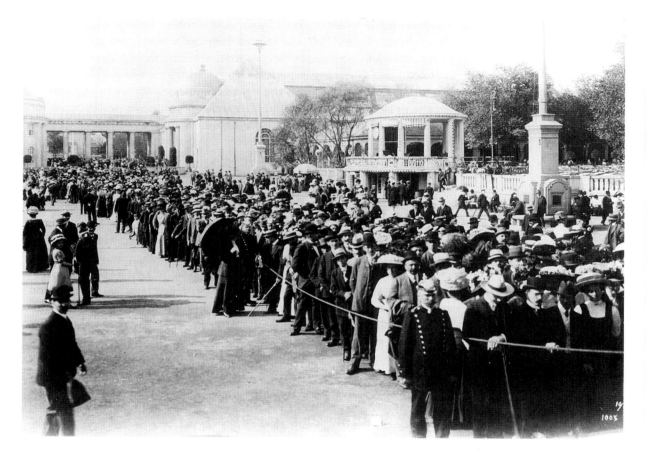

Figure 1. Rush of visitors at the pavilion Man *at the First International Hygiene Exhibition, 1911.*

Werner Spalteholz (1862–1940) had developed a process by which organs could be made transparent or translucent and stained in various colours.[19] The process is based on dehydration of the removed organs and use of an optically transparent embedding material that has the same refractive index as the tissue of the organ itself. Extensive studies were of course needed for this.[20] The transparency and plasticity of the Spalteholz preparations are remarkable even by today's standards. They avoid evoking in the layperson the distaste that is stimulated by moist preparations. The preparations also acquire an almost unearthly radiant appearance when lighting is used to good effect.

Further novelties, each one a superb little technical masterpiece showing the way in which the organs of the human body function in "transparent" working models, were just as exciting. True to Lingner's principle that, without visible demonstration, the explanatory power of words is worth little, the transparent models made lively and comprehensible such complicated interconnections as the circulation of the blood: the arterial and venous systems were shown on a large diagrammatic model, and attached to this was a 365-litre glass tank containing the quantity of blood circulated in half an hour. The pressure that the cardiac muscle has to overcome could be experienced by pressing a rubber ball on a liquid-filled glass tube (*see* Figure 2).[21] The transparency and three-dimensional realism of the Spalteholz preparation remain striking today; for the layperson there is none of that alienating impression left by organs conventionally preserved in a liquid medium and, with the right illumination, the organs actually glow with an almost supernatural iridescence. These novel processes and models offered the layperson a means of understanding the interior of the human body. They were the antithesis of the anatomy room, which had a tendency to affect the senses more than the intellect. Free of bodily, sensual and transient emotions, these carefully designed models bore witness to a faith in the possibility of attaining a state of health and well-being.[22]

The "Gesolei" 1926 – The Transparent Man

The great exhibition of 1911 had two lasting effects. First, its enormous success led to the aspiration of a permanent exhibition, a museum, and second, this first international hygiene exhibition became a model for similar endeavours in later years. Thus, in 1914, Stuttgart hosted an exhibition dedicated to public health care, with the active participation of the then National Hygiene Museum. After the First World War, health and social care exhibitions demonstrated the improved methods of therapy then available to the war disabled. Weapons of mass destruction, trench warfare and poison gas had resulted in an enormous number of disfigurements, amputations and bodily impairments. Apart from improved therapy, the re-integration of the wounded became an important issue in the politically unstable German society after the War.[23]

The true heir of the 1911 exhibition, in size and importance, was the 1926 "Gesolei" ("_Gesundheitspflege, Soziale Fürsorge und Leibesübungen_," perhaps better rendered as "Hesobo" – the care of Health, Social Concern, Bodily Fitness). Thanks to the initiative of the medical doctor Arthur Schloßman and the co-operation of the architect Wilhelm Kreis, an exhibition of ambitious scope had been put in place in Düsseldorf.[24] A substantial proportion of the exhibits was furnished by the German Hygiene Museum. That museum, which was in the initial stages of construction, lent 22 furniture vanfulls of exhibits. The Dresden partners in the exhibition venture assumed responsibility for the core section, *Man*, which, in turn, centred on the subsection *The Transparent Man*. The Dresden museum was concerned to achieve ever more effective techniques of presentation:

It deserves to be emphasised that today's museum's exhibits are based on techniques that differ substantially from those that supported the 1911 Dresden Hygiene Exhibition. Continuing development of means for presentation accelerates obsolescence of hygiene museum exhibits more rapidly than is experienced in other museum fields. Furthermore, account has to be taken of recent advances in scientific research. This imposes curatorial responsibilities for continual review of existent exhibits, their supplementation or modification. The current exhibits therefore comprise relatively few that date back to 1911.[25]

Martin Vogel, Scientific Director of the German Hygiene Museum, had been seconded to co-operate in the planning of the Gesolei exhibition. For Vogel, the continuity between the exhibition on *Man* in Dresden in 1911 and the subsection on *The Transparent Man* in the Gesolei of 1926 was obvious.

As the Transparent Man first came to be "re-awakened" in 1921, it could not be denied that age had already taken its toll and that he could no longer escape critical contemporary review. Since that time, however, he has benefited from continuous recovery, rejuvenation, and growth, and in this process he has evolved in the fashion of a truly well-adapted organism. The enthusiasm of the inspired exhibition-concept creator has indeed linked the medium intimately to the message, the exhibition of the model of man, to man. Our new and most recent jewel in the crown is the "Transparent Man." For the first time, he is now being presented in Düsseldorf to a wide public. The name is no wordplay for here, indeed, the individual organs of man are being presented in such a manner that they can be viewed right through different kinds of tissue, through the bones themselves, and through the blood vessels right down to the finest branchings.[26]

Apart from the technical perfection of the methods of preparation of individual organs, it is the *mise-en-scène* of the Transparent Man that

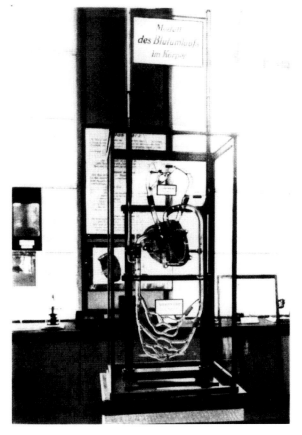

Figure 2. Blood circulation model, 1911. Reproduction Volker Kreidler

impresses so greatly. Notwithstanding his fascination with the attainments of technology, Vogel never lost sight of the totality:

Starting with the functions of the organism and of the organs, the museum's exhibits aim to bring about an understanding of the human body as a whole and in its parts, and in a deeper sense the still inadequately understood importance of the laws of organic life for individual and social conduct of living. In particular, the collection "man" presents much material that is relevant in this context, but other special sections, for instance "propagation, inheritance, and racial hygiene" are conducive to recognition of the same important insights.[27]

The first exhibition dealing with racial hygiene had taken place the year before, from September to December 1925. Building on the ideas of Darwin, Spencer and Galton, eugenics teaching had found a lively response even in socialist and progressive circles. In Britain and the USA too, eugenic themes were widely propagated and were the subject of numerous exhibitions. Independently of Galton, in Germany Alfred Ploetz had developed the concept of "race hygiene," founding a society in 1905.[28]

Man as Prototype of Organisation

The Gesolei presentation of Transparent Man represents the culmination of a vision and of its technical realisation that can be traced back to the ideas of Lingner. A self-made man and successful entrepreneur, Lingner had promoted his visions of health-care enlightenment not merely for their own sake, but always in the context of their value for society as a whole. His credo was summarised in the title of his address when he received an Honorary Doctorate from Bern University: "Man as Prototype of Organisation."[29] The aim of health care is always the smooth functioning of all the organs of the system "man," just as the functioning of the parts of the system "factory" or "state" is a condition for the maintenance and development of those complex systems. In this, Lingner did not proceed from the assumption of an egalitarian-democratic commonality, but from that of a hierarchical ordering.

In a logically ordered system of division of labour, particular organs were therefore the recipients of commands. On this basis, the organisational model of the human organism was equally applicable to Lingner's domain of "the factory." In his manufacturing operations, Lingner placed reliance on new techniques and new technical developments, he was also a pioneer of methods and principles of scientific work organisation, including the conveyor belt, time study and piecework payment. In popular interpretation, the man–machine analogy found its expression in representation of the human digestion system as a factory and, moreover, specific products of the German hygiene museums that seized upon the technique of the Transparent Man and applied it to technical representations: the "Transparent Engine" and the "Transparent Factory." Lingner may not have been the inventor of the man–state or man–factory analogies but, as entrepreneur, he stressed the long-term financial savings and advantages that enlightenment about a healthy and "rational" lifestyle could bring about for the benefit of state, economy and communities.

Presentation in the German Hygiene Museum

In the immediate wake of the successful First International Hygiene Exhibition, consideration had been given to the establishment of an important and central national hygiene museum in Dresden. Oskar von Miller, founder of the Deutsches Museum in Munich, was a committed advocate. When the great exhibition was coming to its end, space had been rented for storage of the great number of exhibits from all the participating nations, and there were also some, perhaps more rudimentary, exhibition areas available for smaller specialty shows. Expectation of an early re-opening of the exhibition stimulated the creation of studios and workshops for the production of exhibits for the museum, and totally new developments through a novel approach to the ideas of transparency. "There was a continuing urge to advance comprehensibility of the structural complexity of the human body. For instance, organs were micro-sliced, each slice individually encapsulated between glass plates, the whole then assembled and bound in book form, so that, in a manner of speaking, the organ could be leafed through."[30]

However, the German Hygiene Museum (after 1918 no longer the National Hygiene Museum) still remained without adequate accommodation. These circumstances were to change only after the museum had participated in the Gesolei. Then, at last, and after the requisite financial resources had been obtained, Wilhelm Kreis, architect of the Düsseldorf exhibition complex, was charged with planning a new building for the German Hygiene Museum in Dresden.

Throughout the period of waiting for a final museum building, the development of attractive models and techniques of display had continued. Valuable experience had been gained in the utilisation of a new plastic known as "Cellon."[31] "One can obtain this material in totally translucent form, in varying degrees of opacity, and in any imaginable colour, one can form its surface to any desired shape, it can be sculpted, drilled, sawn, or milled, one can melt it, press it, blow it like glass, etc., in short one can do anything with it."[32]

Franz Tschakert, Creator of the Transparent Statues

These characteristics of Cellon were familiar to Franz Tschakert, employed by the museum from 1913 till 1925 as "preparer" and after 1925 as chief of the Cellon section in the museum. Around 1926, Tschakert attempted a totally new kind of statue-model; while he does not appear to have left any personal account of this, we do have one from a witness at the time.[33] The birthplace of the statue was not actually the museum itself, but a little closet in a small Dresden enterprise, the manufacturers of almonds,

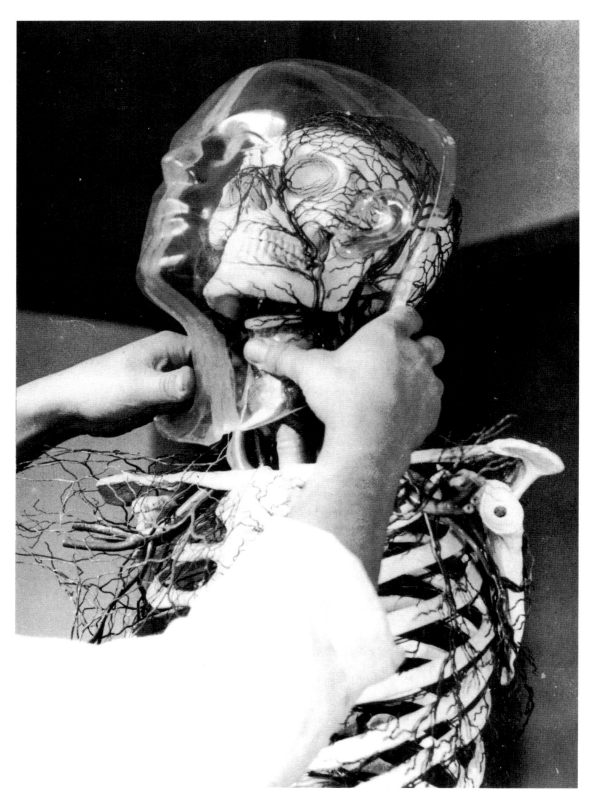

Figure 3. Applying the Cellon skin.

preserves and marmalade, Siemank & Ringelhahn. Tschakert had been friendly with Ringelhahn, who let him have the space, equipped with a steam line, required for the shaping of the Cellon parts. To begin with, Tschakert managed to obtain a human skeleton that he endowed, under the eyes of inquisitive neighbouring children and with the help of some wires and supports, with an erect stature. Next, the skeleton had to be given a human appearance. For that, "Jumbo" was stuffed with wood chips and covered with layers of gypsum until he had attained a human shape. "Gipsumjumbo" then served Tschakert for production of a multi-part mould. Each part was closed with a lid, then, between lid and form, Tschakert inserted a sheet of celluloid that could be subjected to steam pressure via the lid and heated, softened and forced into the mould by the steam pressure. After subsequent water cooling, a moulding of the exterior shape could be withdrawn from the form. This could be cut, and the different parts glued together. The arms, legs, parts of the torso, etc. could then all be put together around the skeleton, in dismountable manner.[34] The inner organs were derived from wax models in a nearby school where the director was a friend of Tschakert's. The organs were thus formed in the same manner as the exterior body, and afterwards they were painted according to their original colours. Finally, the system of blood vessels was represented in red for arteries and blue for veins, and supplemented by the principal nerves, portrayed in green (see Figure 3).

Tschakert found a growing interest among the curators and management of the museum. When the statue was completed, awaiting only completion of the exterior skin, Werner Spalteholz (inventor of the aforementioned transparent organs) was invited to make an appraisal. "He was astonished and enthusiastic when he saw the statue. He had never imagined the feasibility of such perfection and attainment of scientific exactitude."[35] Eventually, Tschakert and his almost completed statue were able to leave his rudimentary workshop and move to the museum workshops. In June 1927, the Board of Trustees examined "a newly constructed model, 'Man as a Prime Example of Technical Perfection,'" although, pending patent applications, it was not yet to be exhibited.[36] Construction of the transparent statue was finally completed in the museum workshops.

As an artisan, Tschakert had achieved an advance that the scientists within the museum had held to be desirable, but had not themselves been able to achieve: the transition from the presentation of individual organs to a model that presented all essential parts of the body in their true positions, in functional relation, and within a complete body. Tschakert may be seen as having been truly predestined for this achievement, for he had joined the museum within the lifetime of Lingner, and had become manager of the Cellon workshops. With his expertise in the handling of this versatile material, he was more capable than anyone else of building, first the parts, and then the complete human body.

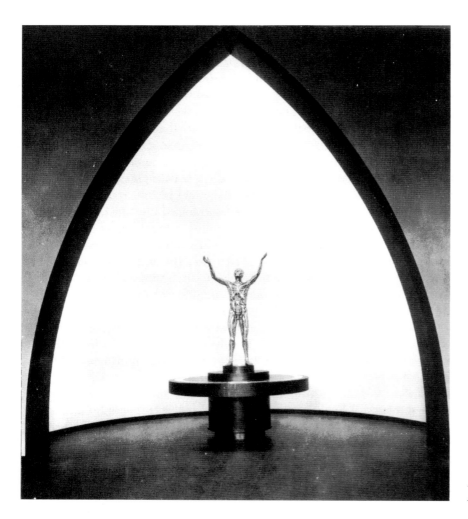

Figure 4. The Transparent Man, 1930.

The Grand Opening – the Transparent Man, the New Museum,
and Second International Hygiene Exhibition

The first Transparent Man was to be unveiled on a special occasion, underlining its importance to the management of the German Hygiene Museum. After many years during which the museum had functioned only in temporary premises, complemented by mobile exhibitions, the management had at last succeeded in gaining the combined support of the German State, the Federal State of Saxony and the town of Dresden in financing the museum. The foundation stone was laid on October 7 and 8, 1927. Two years later, the staff moved into the new premises. Only a few months remained in which to fill the galleries with exhibition material, and to organise the Second International Hygiene Exhibition in Dresden, to be held within the grounds of the museum to mark its official opening.

The museum itself was an impressive building, with congress and exhibition halls around an inner courtyard. Fronted by two towers flanking the impressive colonnade of the main building, the museum measured 100 × 160 metres, and the main building reached a height of 29 metres. Part of the inner courtyard was covered, and contained the central exhibition *Man*. Above all, the position of the museum was made impressive through its location on the kilometre-long access from the "great garden," an enormous landscaped garden containing Dresden's first baroque buildings, which cut through the centre of the museum. On that transept through the museum, Wilhelm Kreis had erected sculptures by two other German academicians. A little further along that main axis, he had added an apse, almost a chapel to *Man*, as the site of the museum's chief attraction, a unique masterpiece: the Transparent Man. On May 16, 1930, the portals of the museum opened for the first time. The hopes that accompanied the opening of the new institution were expressed in deeply moving terms by Oskar von Miller, who concluded his inauguration speech with the words: "I hope that the Hygiene Museum will see the day when a man at my age of 75 years shall no longer be seen as a well-preserved old man of hoary years, but as one still in alert youth."[37]

The Career of a Principle: *The Transparent Man* in the Period of National Socialism

In Exalted Posture – the "Adoration of the Sun" as an Ideal

The symbolism of the model was expressed by its position within the inner sanctum of the museum, by its bearing, and finally by the material itself. Bruno Gebhard, who had been scientific collaborator in the setting up of the museum, refers to an illustrious prototype of the figure, the Greek statue "Adoring Youth," that is ascribed to Boedas of Byzantium (*c.* 300 BC). In fact, the fine arts of the nineteenth and twentieth centuries have long been influenced by the model of the erect figure with outstretched arms. That prayer stance (erect, arms bent or stretched out, palms open, gaze directed obliquely upward) conveys to the viewer, even to one not versed in the canons of religious gesture, a consciousness of appeal to the superhuman-divine. The same stance had been adopted by the adherents of new life reform movements in the first decades of the twentieth century. In the "light adoration" the unclothed body is turned to the sun, in expectation of a this-worldly health bestowed by light and air, while at the same time striving to overcome the here and now in conscious appeal to the sun as salvation, in place of a rejected, traditional deity that is to be sloughed off with its bourgeois society and customs.[38]

It is not only the posture of our statue that is designed to overcome corporeality, with its association of uncleanliness; it is, above all, the vitreous figure, the transparency. The individual characteristics of an individual's appearance – skin and hair, muscle and fat – are all missing in the Transparent Man. He is transparent right through; nothing remains hidden. The figure firstly symbolises, in utmost clarity, the claims of an unchallenged natural science that believes itself bound less and less by any secrets, and secondly, it belongs to the aesthetic school of the Bauhaus, which even the monument-inclined Wilhelm Kreis could not escape, and which is responsible for the most successful aspects of its buildings. The elimination of all ornamentation, and a striving for clarity and transparency were principles which the directors of the Bauhaus (originally in Weimar, then from 1926 as the State College in Dessau) carried through in their aesthetic programme, from architecture, via fashion, to the construction of industrially manufactured everyday articles. The distinguished architect Walter Gropius, for example, designed the door-latches for the German Hygiene Museum. The architectonic style of the Bauhaus found its continuation and worldwide extension in the "International Style."

The fact that the Transparent Man is not made of glass, but of a plastic, has endowed him over the years with an unexpected, although very human, quality, namely that of ageing. Thus the oldest preserved models, of the size of a present-day 12- to 14-year-old, appear, when removed from their plinths, fragile, almost in need of protection. The skin of the plastic has lost its cool lustre, which has given way to a warmer tone; the transparency is diminished and almost hides the inner organs. To the people of the time, however, the figure was in many ways a symbol: for the claims of modern natural science in understanding and explanation of complex connections; for a transparency that, in its attitude of adoration, achieved a transcendency; and, finally, for a time that aimed, through rationality and enlightenment, to dislodge traditional social and aesthetic conventions. The fact that the German Hygiene Museum continues, to this day, to be regarded as a temple of hygiene, appears to confirm the symbolic power of the unusual exhibit.

Transparent Figures – German Achievement of Quality

After the successful inauguration of the vitreous man on the occasion of the opening of the museum buildings, the model became a star attraction of numerous special exhibitions. Interest had awakened, not only in Germany but in numerous countries abroad. One high point in the attainments of Berlin exhibitions before the Second World War was doubtlessly the display *The Miracle of Life*. The German Hygiene Museum sent Bruno Gebhard to Berlin, where he organised the show covering an area of 40,000 square metres (approx. 400,000 square feet) around the Berlin Radio Tower. It was Gebhard's aim to "achieve health education with visual methods." The design can be described as modern even today: for example, the entire 3,200 square metres (approx. 32,000 square feet) of the ceiling of one hall was painted bright red, in order to demonstrate the surface area of the red blood corpuscles of a single person. The most modern methods of visualisation, such as the so-called "microvivaria" – microscopes with projection facilities that could demonstrate the propagation of single

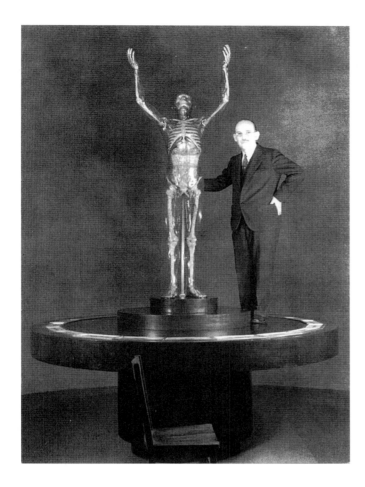

Figure 5. The Transparent Man in the Buffalo Museum of Science, 1934.

cells – stood out alongside others of unrefined nationalist pathos. The chief attraction, again, was the Transparent Man.

An International Success

The "German Achievement of Quality" found admirers beyond the frontiers of the country, for example at the Paris World Exhibition of 1937. A complete pavilion was provided here for the "Homme de Verre" and attracted such a flood of visitors that it had to remain open well into the night.[39] Greater even than that in Europe was the admiration (and market) for the Transparent Man in the USA, as was also the case for *Eugenics in the New Germany*. The German Hygiene Museum had an exhibition on that theme in 1934–35 in Los Angeles, in Portland and in Salem, Oregon, and finally also in Buffalo, New York. In Buffalo, the Museum of Science now also hosted the exhibit of a further statue from Dresden (*see* Figure 5).[40]

The strong US export market was sustained by the American infrastructure surrounding the popularisation of science and health education. After 1930 there were close contacts with the American Public Health Organisation, which counted some 10,000 members. In 1934, members of this organisation invited the German Hygiene Museum to participate in an annual exhibition. The Americans proposed, and the Germans accepted, the theme of *Eugenics in the New Germany*.[41] Existing international contacts and a certain admiration for the choreographic attainments of German exhibition organisers prepared the way for the triumphant tours of the transparent men through the United States. The donors of the "Transparent Woman" advertised themselves in the trade publication of the underwear manufacturers: "'Know thyself' has now become a scientific possibility for every woman. By seeing herself in the transparent woman, she can gain an appreciation of the value of medical science, and with this information on the mechanism of her body, she can learn how to guide its well-being and control and correct its appearance."[42]

There is no exact information about the number of transparent people that were made before 1945. We can, however, deduce from the diverse sources available, a rough history of the careers of the following statues:

- Franz Tschakert's first creation was shown in the German Hygiene Museum from 1930 onwards. It was totally destroyed in 1945.
- A statue was made for the World Exhibition of 1933 in Chicago, and has since been in the Mayo Medical Museum in Rochester, New York.
- After 1934, the Buffalo Museum of Science exhibited the figure that has already been referred to. As an outcome of research for a joint exhibition of the German Hygiene Museum and the German Historical Museum, *Visitations of the Body. Views of the Body in Five Centuries*, Dresden 1990, the figure came into the possession of the German Historical Museum in Berlin, where it remains today.
- For the design of the Berlin Exhibition *Miracle of Life*, a figure was specially made, and was later shown in many repertory exhibitions. It was probably this figure that was also to be seen in post-1945 repertory exhibitions.
- Another figure that was exhibited to a wide public had been produced for a 1936 exhibition in Stockholm under the theme "Mother and Child," and was also shown in 1937–38 at the World Exhibition in Paris. The figure then began a migration throughout Europe; it was shown in Madrid in 1944, but nothing further is known about its whereabouts since that time.
- It is claimed, although there are no official records, that there was another female figure that was shown in the USA in connection with the presentation of corsetry. This may refer to a Transparent Woman, donated by the corsetry manufacturer, S. H. Kemp of Jackson, Missouri. After first showing in 1936 in the New York Museum of Science and

Industry, that model, which was also known as "Miss Science" migrated through shows in 100 towns of the USA and ended in the Science Centre in St Louis, Missouri. Like the model from Buffalo, this model is today in the possession of the German Historical Museum, Berlin, and is exhibited on loan in the German Hygiene Museum in Dresden.

- A Transparent Man was made in 1937 for a museum in the Japanese town of Nagoya. No further details are known of it.
- Another model was made in 1937 for the USA, on the order of the Oberland Trust and the Carl Schurz Memorial Trust, and was shown for several years in a hygiene touring exhibition. Nothing is known of its fate after it reached Texas.
- Even during the War, under difficult conditions, work progressed in the German Hygiene Museum on another Transparent Man. Essential parts had been stored in a cellar and survived bomb attacks, to provide parts-support for post-war production.

The Transparent Principle: Transparent Engine, Transparent Factory

The success of the Transparent Man led to an enthusiasm for its explanatory principle. There was an attempt to render other complex connections transparently demonstrable. Thus the Auto Union AG in Chemnitz commissioned the Plexiglas Workshops of the German Hygiene Museum to make a transparent engine. A full-sized, 2.7 litre, six-cylinder engine was made in Dresden and shown at the motor exhibition of 1938 in Berlin (*see* Figure 6). It is not easy to demonstrate to a layperson the sequence of events within an internal combustion engine, but the new techniques of transparent modelling permitted a ready explanation of the normally invisible combustion stages. In the same way that the Transparent Man was a purely transparent creation, without fleshiness or scent, without fat or muscle, so also the transparent motor could be devoid of petrol, hot oil, cooling waters and combustion products, heat and violent movement. The transparent engine remained a unique creation. In 1945, Soviet troops took it to Moscow to the Polytechnic Museum.

The attractiveness of the principle in demonstrating technical connections had now been well confirmed and was extended in a Transparent Factory. It is not known who prepared the draft designs for this lavish model; however, Tschakert, the Museum's Workshop Manager, certainly had some responsible involvement in its production. The entire model was a work commissioned for the *Healthy Living – Happy Production* Exhibition held in Berlin in 1938. New ideas were presented on a larger scale.

Why "Transparent Factory"? Health and the ability to work are the most precious possessions of the German people. The recognition that everything must be done to conserve and promote them, gains more and more acceptance, and gives assurance that enterprises take all requisite measures … This method of fabrication of transparent

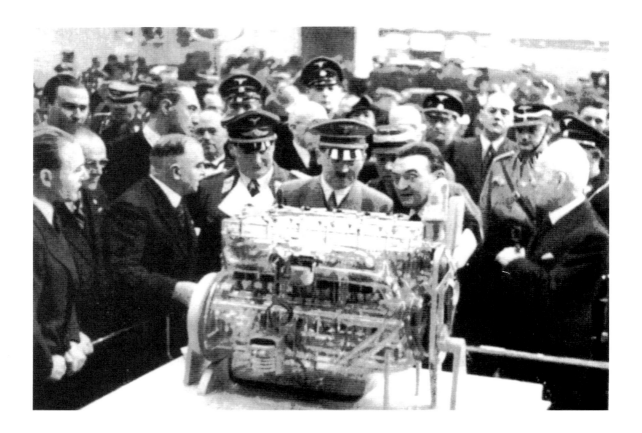

Figure 6. Hitler and Göring at the viewing of the Transparent Engine at the Berlin Car Show, 1938. Reproduction Volker Kreidler

models is now also to be employed in the service of propaganda for factory hygiene. The model of a factory was designed with walls made of the German synthetic material "Plexiglas." Like the Transparent Man, the model was manufactured in the experienced workshops of the German Hygiene Museum.[43]

Like the model Man a few years earlier, the Transparent Factory gained renown as a masterpiece. The details were indeed impressive. Manufactured to a scale of $1:15$, 6 metres high, with a diameter of 8 metres, a total weight of 1250 kg, assembled with 3000 screws, 1½ km of electric wiring, made in 2850 hours, and rendered transparent through 107 square metres of the new synthetic, Plexiglas, it could be rotated for presentation to the viewer.

The factory model is designed to give the viewer the impression of a well-ordered mechanism. It is not a question of working time, of profit or loss; the factory appears as an organic whole that has been optimised for the preservation of health and work as the acclaimed highest of objectives. The factory is no Moloch, does not frighten; rather it is light, and equipped with all facilities, inclusive of a sports stadium. Sweat and smoking chimneys do not exist in this ideal factory, any more than blood courses through the veins of the Transparent Man. Lingner's thesis of man as an organising principle finds its highest expression in the Transparent Factory – in a state in which a virtual reality of propaganda whitewashed the factory organisation of a whole state, including the factory-like removal of all undesirables.

New Edition of a Successful Product: Transparent Man in Post-War Germany

New Beginning in Dresden

Even in the final years of the Second World War and of National Socialism, the German Hygiene Museum continued with its exhibitions. Apart from racial propaganda, and in spite of the environment of crisis and the advance of the allies, there were also non-political themes designed to suggest the existence of a kind of normality and of the everyday world – for instance a "sauna exhibition" was opened on June 18, 1944.

Immediately after the arrival of Soviet troops in Dresden, the German Hygiene Museum was subordinated to the Soviet military administration. In parallel with the operations to clear up the destroyed museum building, the completion of a preserved Transparent Man was energetically pursued, for it was intended as early as October 1945 that the supervision of the museum was to pass from the occupational administration to the new German Central Administration for Health, then the Soviet Zone of Occupation. A celebration on November 23, 1946 was the first occasion for the Museum to demonstrate a newly created transparent figure and explain the scope for future work. Dr Neubert, appointed as Director in March 1946, explained the threads linking past and present:

The Hygiene Museum does not aim at fixed prescriptions, it will not give superficial instruction, it will aim to mediate a profound knowledge of man, so that every individual may participate with personal understanding in the ordinances of the health authorities. Thus deeper understanding will teach people to distinguish between the genuine and the phoney, the true needs of men and the superficial stimulants of advertisements. It teaches a proper ranking of needs and therefore leads straight to the planned economy, or, in other words, to socialism.[44]

However, the positive advances of a planned economy were not yet quite in evidence, and the production of the first Transparent Man of the post-war era was characterised by expediency: a wooden plinth had to take the place of a metal plinth, and in view of the expense of frosted glass, window glass had to be frosted by hand.

Competition in the West

This first post-war Transparent Man was not the only representative of its species, for there had been another figure touring in Western Germany during the years preceding the War's end, and in November 1946 the authorities in Dresden learned, through a former prisoner of war who had been held in Schleswig-Holstein (an American zone of occupation), that a German Hygiene Museum statue had been found there, in the attic of a farm in the neighbourhood of Eutin.[45] That was no great surprise to the museum. One Johannes Erler had been in the employ of the museum as manager of external touring exhibitions until May 1944. In correspondence between Erler and Dresden in October 1945, instructions from Dresden for the return of a statue to Dresden had been evasively answered, and Erler eventually began his own exhibition activity in Kiel and Lübeck, with the implicit permission of the museum.

The post-war inauguration of the Transparent Man in West Germany may thus be seen to date from the beginning of July 1946 in Kiel. In the face of considerable difficulties, Erler wandered through various towns, carefully observed from a distance by the German Hygiene Museum. At the beginning of 1950, he arrived with his exhibit in Cologne, and had it brought up to date in the hygienic-anatomical laboratories of the Office for Health Affairs. This signified the beginning of the end of the activities of the Dresden Museum in West Germany, for these laboratories were already under the authority of the newly established German Health Museum in Cologne.

Erler found support for his activity in Cologne. Georg Seiring, the President of the German Hygiene Museum who had entered into its service in 1913 when Lingner was still alive, and who had also been in charge of the museum during the Nazi period, had emigrated to West Germany with a considerable number of colleagues, including Franz Tschakert.[46] There, in Cologne, a new German Health Museum was to be founded, modelled on the Dresden original. In addition to permanent exhibitions, the proven success of touring exhibitions was to be continued, and a health academy was to train teachers in matters of health care. Furthermore, the production of educational material and of models was also to be restarted in Cologne, and with it that of the Transparent Man. From January 1950, they toured the Dresden-made statue that had been part of Johann Erler's touring exhibits.

While, in Dresden, conditions had changed, Seiring and his colleagues were immediately able to resume their pre-war contacts. It is therefore not surprising that the first statue from Cologne, after an exhibition in London, found its final destination in the Health Museum in Cleveland, Ohio. A snide, if not quite accurate, comment was addressed to former Dresden colleagues: "The Transparent Man from Dresden has emigrated to Moscow. Now a new generation is departing from Cologne to the Western world."[47] The formerly proud symbol of German health education had become a bone of contention in East–West conflict.[48]

The Eastern world reacted to the Cologne provocation with socialist indignation under the title "Western Lies about the Transparent Woman:"

These defamations by the West are too obvious to disguise their true intent. The staff of the German Hygiene Museum raise their voice in protest and respond with strengthened resolution for improved performance and heightened quality, in dedication to a peaceful, united, and democratic all-Germany.[49]

An Excursion to Moscow

The promising expectation of a new generation of transparent men did in reality have a greater chance of realisation in Moscow. A Dresden "Transparent Couple" travelled to Moscow; not abducted, but presented to the brotherly Occupation Power. In response to a proposal by the personnel of the German Hygiene Museum, the government of the State of Saxony had passed a formal resolution to that effect in December 1949. The statues were to cost around 80,000 Marks. The occasion was not an unimportant one: the statues were to be presented to "Generalissimus Stalin for his 70th birthday as a token of the quality of achievement attainable by co-operation of brawn and brain." On December 15, 1949, the Society for German–Soviet Friendship acknowledged receipt of six dispatch containers; this left just six days for transport and for the organisation required in Moscow in order to meet the date of the birthday on December 21. It is not known how pleased Stalin was with this birthday gift from Dresden.[50] The Transparent Couple was eventually to be displayed to the Soviet people in travelling exhibitions.[51]

It was not clear, either, whether this gift was totally spontaneous, or whether it was an imposed, if delayed, reparation. For the observer of today, however, the Transparent Couple seems to perfectly symbolise Stalin's concept of new man. A tightly organised existence within the State and the economy that imposes a socialist lifestyle right down to the minutiae of privacy, is perfectly represented by the Transparent Man in his ambivalence. He represents life not as it is, but as the victory of science over the imperfection of individuality; he represents the negation of corporeality that, like all individuality, obstructs thorough organisation. Above all, the Transparent Man shows that there is nothing to hide, that the last darkness has been removed, and that nothing can be kept from the devotees of such symbols. That, of all occasions, the Transparent Woman and the Transparent Man were to be joined on the occasion of a Stalin birthday celebration, can also be taken as signifying the transparency of even the private life of interaction and intimacy, even of its dissolution in favour of the creation of a new generation that is only aware of the supremacy of society.

Socialist Production I: A New Transparent Man

Early objectives, envisaged since the First International Hygiene Exhibition in 1911, for economic support of the German Hygiene Museum through production and marketing of high-class exhibition materials and models for the advancement of health education, were again realised by Georg Seiring in Cologne. The price of the transparent figure that was sold to Cleveland was 50,000 Marks; nevertheless, the growing production of Transparent

Men in Dresden during the years after 1950, in the face of continuing problems of shortage of materials cannot be explained exclusively in terms of expectations of profit, especially as a substantial proportion of the figures were delivered to socialist brother countries. Instead, the Transparent Man served the consciously promoted self-confidence of the East German State that elevated it above an article of commerce to a symbol of the truly socialist state that, for the first time, devoted itself seriously – and above all more intensively than the capitalist countries – to the objectives of popular health education. In addition to sales, therefore, there were gifts: to comrade Stalin, to institutions of needy allied countries, and to the World Health Organisation. On the occasion of the 26th Congress of the WHO in 1974, East Germany, always concerned about its international reputation, donated a Transparent Woman, still to be seen there, to the Geneva office of the Organization. The Health Minister, Mecklinger, was saluted by the heads of the WHO.

The everyday problems of East Germany, an economy characterised by material shortages, stood in contrast to the image presented in public. One episode in the history of the Cold War was mirrored in the museum's production of its model. Despite Ulbricht's claim that no one intended to erect a wall, the government directed an enquiry to the Dresden Hygiene Museum on August 8, 1961 in relation to "dependence of our production on imports, and steps taken to correct it."[52] Whereas raw materials needed for building the Berlin Wall after August 13, 1961 could be obtained without difficulty, there were problems in procuring plastics. Stocks of Cellon were not large, and hence production of the Transparent Man had to be changed to use of the East German plastic, Piacryl. However, the special adhesive required to glue Piacryl was still obtainable only from West Germany. The resolution of these technological problems must be attributed to a recognition by the East German government that the Dresden institution was not just a constituent of the nation's health system, but an important factor in its economy too.

Socialist Production II: Transparent Animals
Notwithstanding supply difficulties, the transparent figures had become articles of value and were widely exported. Available records show that, between 1945 and 1997, a total of 114 statues were manufactured and sold – 67 Women and 47 Men. Whilst the range of transparent products had been supplemented during the National Socialist time by an engine and a factory, this range was now widened by two of the most important domesticated animals: the cow and the horse. A ministerial letter dated June 2, 1950 asked for initiation of the production of a "Transparent Horse" and a "Transparent Cow". The request reflected practical motives.[53] Growing rationalisation of agriculture in East Germany called for a core of well-trained experts that needed to be supported by adequate educational aids. The need for foreign currencies, procurable through exports, may have

been equally relevant. The ambitious project was, however, delayed for years by shortages of expertise, so that the inauguration did not take place until June 2, 1956, in the presence of the Health Minister, Luipold Streidle, during the 750th anniversary celebrations of the town of Dresden.

Production had been taken in hand with great care and with the co-operation of diverse scientific institutes. The original proportions of the animals in question had been minutely observed, and their realisation represented a remarkable scientific, technical and artistic achievement. After 1959, the Dresden product range constituted almost a glazed Noah's ark. These were not the fantasy products of their creators, who in the last resort were also their marketeers; the transparent animals had been created through substantial efforts and at costs that might have been harder to justify under the principles of a market economy, but were intended as new and important objects of symbolism in a state that also organised its agriculture according to rational, factory-inspired principles. The worldwide uniqueness of the figures, combined with their high visual attractiveness, secured for East Germany a high reputation, particularly in countries that were technically less developed and had emerging economies and a predominance of agriculture.

The Legend Lives

Today, there are still transparent figures in the German Hygiene Museum. Many visitors ask first at the ticket desk, not for the current special exhibits that the museum mounts in considerable numbers, but for the location of the Transparent Woman. She stands, as in the display of earlier years, in a kind of temple, although today's visitors no longer have to stand in admiration, for an amphitheatre of benches is provided for an audio lecture. Within its staged setting, the model continues to evoke an astonishment that is quite incomparable to that of, say, an X-ray picture.

It is unimaginable that a visitor to the Museum would miss the statues, and certainly none would wish to miss the reactions of nostalgic visitors. The Transparent Man remains an effective, well-designed model for the graphic presentation of the basic principles of human anatomy.

The marketing of the Transparent Man has not ceased. The interests of the museum no longer centre on the attainment of volume output, however. It aims to retain its fund of experience and the technical know-how of the people who make the models, but the statues' uniqueness to Dresden is to be emphasised, and so sales within Europe have stopped. Enquiries for transparent men are numerous; videos are made, particularly for TV productions with medical or humanistic-scientific contexts; museums and major specialty exhibitions frequently approach the museum requesting loans of the statues. The museum has two "travel figures" available for this last requirement. However, all enquiries are critically reviewed, to avoid excessive exposure of the figures and of their reproductions.[54]

The Competition

Can the Transparent Man, with his perhaps now old-fashioned technology and aesthetic presentation, not to mention the burden of his symbolic significance, compete in any way with other media? These are now numerous, and only a few can be mentioned here. The fascination of a view into the human body has become a very high-tech, high-cost, difficult-to-manage system of image production. Ever since the development of X-ray technology for medical diagnosis and treatment, the use of modern imaging techniques has become indispensable for popular scientific demonstrations. Apart from the well-established X-ray systems, since the 1970s there has been computed tomography [CT], now supplemented by positron emission tomography [PET], which enables a view of biochemical processes. Another development offering great prospects is magnetic resonance imaging [MRI]. Furthermore, according to the experts, truly novel insights may be gained from a combination of methods, for example an imaging process in combination with brain scanning [electroencephalography, EEG]. Thus it is probable that, not

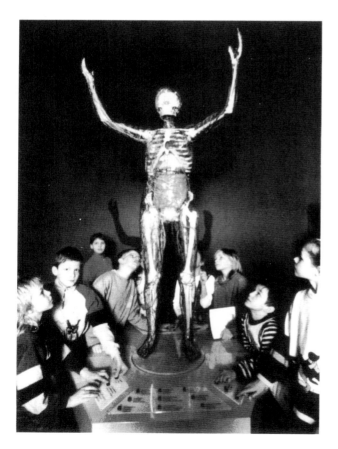

Figure 7. Young visitors with the Transparent Woman, 1997. Photograph André Rival

only the anatomy of the body, but also its inner dynamics will be opened to view – a radical advance in the observation of the interior of the human body.

The other side of the coin of the flood of information is the problem of its administration. It is said that the image archive of a large hospital grows by a cubic metre each day.[55] Still more pictures stem from computers with great capacities that are capable of transforming images into totally new, dynamic, three-dimensional views. This technique can create pictures of high aesthetic appeal, some of which have already become classics, such as "Voxel Man" and the "Visible Human Project." The "Virtual Head" from the computer centre of the Hamburg University Clinic has already been reproduced many times in popular scientific magazines. In contrast, the digitalised frozen slices of a corpse, made by the University Clinic of Colorado, have a strange effect on many viewers because they are those of an executed criminal. This does not in any way detract from its fascination, and above all its popularity: like the Hamburg head, the body from Colorado can be viewed on the Internet.[56] Thus, we come full circle from our introductory sentences, for Vesalius also is to be found on the Internet. The father of all anatomy gives his name to a data bank that stores material for specific anatomical views.[57]

Future of a "Wonderwork"
If Vesalius represents a data bank, is the computer-supported sliced man from Colorado the new Transparent Man? At any time and anywhere, he provides a view, not only of essential structures, but of innumerable details. Or, is it the Human Genome Project – which aims to decipher the totality of human genetic material within the next few years – that represents the fulfilment of the wish for a view into the most profound interior? In the face of the wealth of data involved in these projects, of the numbers of scientists who are involved, and of the amounts of money required, these statues have become a relic of scientific history, a fossil of science popularisations. However, it is a property of fossils that, beyond the artefacts themselves, they offer insight to the times of their creation. Thus it is that the Transparent Man, as he appears today in the German Hygiene Museum, is less a popular science-mediating object but rather more a piece of history; he is a unique testimony, not only to the Dresden Museum, but also to concepts of progress, enlightenment and producibility. At the turn of the millennium, in his 70th year, he will thus attain a further pinnacle, for the German Hygiene Museum is preparing a large exhibition section for the World Exhibition, Expo 2000, in Hanover, to be called, as it was 70 years earlier, *Man*. Fascinating new insights of human sciences are to be shown there, and there, too, will be, in all its modesty, the Transparent Man. One thing will become clear within the flood of information: that the true miracle work is not the plastic statue, but Man.

Notes

In approaching this subject, I have relied in the first place on the excellent work of Rosmarie Beier and Martin Roth, who have been the first to deal historically-critically with the creation and the repercussions of this unique model. Hearty thanks also go to Barbara Köster, who edited the article. A further thank you to Marion Schneider, archivist of the Deutsches Hygiene Museum, for her very helpful research. I am very obliged to Prof. Richard Funk, Institute for Anatomy at the Medical Faculty Carl Gustav Carus, Technical University Dresden, for making it possible to visit the rooms in the Institute and for his numerous explanations. The editors and author are grateful to Martin Bud and Evelyne Draper for translating this article.

1. The German description "Gläserner Mensch" is far better suited to show the symbolic and the quite ambivalent characteristics than the conventional translation "Transparent Man."
2. Rosmarie Beier and Martin Roth, eds., *Der Gläserne Mensch – eine Sensation. Zur Kulturgeschichte eines Ausstellungsobjekts* (Stuttgart, 1990).
3. "Anatomy" is translated from the Greek for "to cut"; today it is only used figuratively as a generic term for the science of the structure of living things. Anatomy explains the structure of the body, the organs, tissues, cells and the organic, and their co-ordination and function. In German, "Sektion" and "Obduktion" are no longer differentiated in everyday language. The Latin "sectio," which is today an established part of the study of medicine, was originally used for the actual opening up of a corpse to diagnose the cause of illness or death. The Latin "obducere" is translated as "to pull something over something." "Obduction" was used for the final covering of the corpse.
4. Quoted from H. Roessler, "Hector Berlioz und seine medizinische Karriere," *Medizinischer Monatsspiegel* 1 (1960): 2.
5. In the last years of his life, Dürer devoted himself to the completion of his theoretical writings: Albrecht Dürer, *Unterweisung der Messung mit Zirkel und Richtscheit in Linien, Ebenen und ganzen Körpern* (Nürnberg, 1525) and Albrecht Dürer, *Vier Bücher von menschlichen Proportionen* (Nürnberg, 1528).
6. Rosmarie Beier, "Der Blick in den Körper. Zur Geschichte des gläsernen Menschen in der Neuzeit," in Beier and Roth, eds. (n. 2 above), p. 14 f.
7. Andreas Vesalius, *De humani corporis fabrica libris septem* (Basel, 1543).
8. Wilhelm Conrad Röntgen, *Eine neue Art von Strahlen* (Würzburg, 1896).
9. Bernike Pasveer, "Knowledge of Shadows: The Introduction of X-ray Images in Medicine," *Sociology of Health and Illness* 11 (1988): 360–81.
10. Octave Mannoni, *Sigmund Freud in Selbstzeugnissen und Bilddokumenten* (Reinbek, 1971); Ernst Freud et al., *Sigmund Freud. Sein Leben in Bildern und Texten* (Frankfurt, 1985).
11. Sigmund Freud, *Gesammelte Werke* (Collected Works), vol. 2/3 (Frankfurt). At the wish of the author the work bears the date "1900."
12. Cf. Gerhard A. Ritter, *Der Sozialstaat. Entstehung und Entwicklung im internationalen Vergleich* (Munich, 1991).
13. For exhibitions in general see, Paul Greenhalgh, *Ephemeral Vistas: The Expositions Universelles, Great Expositions and World Fairs 1851–1939* (Manchester, Eng., 1988). Social-economic and social-hygiene questions had already been raised at the Paris World Exhibition, 1855, within the framework of a "Galerie de l'économie." Martin Vogel, "Hygiene-Ausstellungen und Hygiene-Museen in früherer Zeit," *Hygienischer Wegweiser* 5 (1930): 145 f. The Englishman D. Twining was a leader in endeavours "to set up an economic museum for the working classes." In 1852, he presented his ideas which, however, were not initially realised. Martin Vogel (above), p. 145. Tietze discussed hygiene exhibitions in Leeds (1871), Norwich (1873), Glasgow (1874), Brighton (1875), Liverpool (1876) and London (1881). Particularly noteworthy is the Great Health Exhibition of May 8 to October 30, 1884 in London, which occupied 1,600,000 square feet and attracted over 4 million visitors. Felix Tietze, "Die Internationale Hygiene-Ausstellung London 1884," *Hygienischer Wegweiser* 5 (1930): 149 ff.
14. In greater detail in Martin Roth, "Menschenökonomie oder der Mensch als technisches und künstlerisches Meisterwerk," in Beier and Roth, eds. (n. 2 above), p. 46 ff.
15. Victor Klemperer, *Curriculum Vitae*, ed. von Walter Nowojski (Berlin, 1996), vol. 2, p. 609.
16. Susanne Roeßiger, "In aller Munde – das Deutsche Hygiene-Museum," in *In aller Munde. Einhundert Jahre Odol*, ed. Martin Roth, Manfred Scheske, and Hans-Christian Täubrich (Stuttgart, 1993), p. 52.

17. Karl August Lingner (b. 21 December 1861 in Magdeburg, d. 5 June 1916, Dresden). Trained as a businessman, in 1892 founded Dresden Chemical Laboratory, known after 1898 as Lingner Works. Lingner funded a variety of social initiatives in Dresden: 1897 the Central Laboratory for Dental Health and children's clinic and nursery; 1897 Disinfection centre and public reading room. In 1900 he became a commercial councillor and in 1912 was awarded an honorary doctorate by the University of Bern.

18. Karl August Lingner, "Einige Leitgedanken zu der Sonderausstellung: Volkskrankheiten und ihre Bekämpfung," in *Die deutschen Städte* (Leipzig, 1904), vol. 1, p. 533.

19. Hendrik Behling, *Das anatomische Labor am Deutschen Hygiene-Museum Dresden. Ein Beitrag zur Geschichte der Anatomie in Dresden* (Dresden, 1996), p. 18 ff.

20. Werner Spalteholz, *Über das Durchsichtigmachen von menschlichen und tierischen Präparaten* (Leipzig, 1914), p. 67, cited from Behling (n. 19 above), p. 18, among others: "1. preparation of body/organ (removal of scales, squama, hair, fur, etc.), injection, 2. fixation, 3. possible decalcification, 4. bleaching (with hydrogen peroxide, depending on whether acidic or weakly alkaline), 5. rinse thoroughly with water, 6. dehydration in increasing alcohol concentrations (up to 100%), 7. transfer into benzene (change twice) [fire hazard!], 8. immerse in final liquid, 9. evacuate to remove benzene in the air." (A mixture of bezyl benzoate, Safrol, Isosafrol and oil of Wintergreen was used as embedding fluid.)

21. *Official Catalogue of the International Hygiene Exhibition, Dresden, May to October 1911*. New Improved Edition, Berlin (n.d.), p. 383 ff.

22. The activities of the museum included further processes of preparation and representation of human organs, e.g. a "process for representing blood vessels by injection with a new mixture which chemically destroys the surrounding body tissues;" also, the Spalteholz process was further developed and achieved new results: "Thereby, it turns out that the process achieves particularly interesting results when it is applied to pathologically changed organs," in *Das National-Hygiene-Museum in Dresden in den Jahren 1912–1918* (Dresden, 1919), p. 12.

23. "One could not devise anything more tactless, anything more defeatist ... than this otherwise admirable exhibition, which, if I am not mistaken, travelled through all the German cities. It exhibits and demonstrates everything that was done for the war-disabled, and what should still be done: from the hospital to the home. A major part, therefore, was of a medical nature. Large models illustrated orthopaedic methods: stretching, resting, bandaging – all this was clean and comforting. But one could also see fresh and scarred wounds reproduced in coloured wax pieces, the condition before and after the resection, the transplant, the plastic surgery. For the surgeon, everything was indisputably artistic and edifying, for the lay person much was atrocious." Klemperer (n. 15 above), p. 609.

24. The "Gesolei" (GE–SO–LEI = **Ge**sundheitspflege, **So**ziale Fürsorge und **Lei**besübungen) became a display of superlatives. The large exhibition for hygiene, social welfare and physical education in Dusseldorf was visited by 7.5 million visitors. *GE-SO-LEI. Große Ausstellung Düsseldorf 1926. Für Gesundheitspflege, Soziale Fürsorge und Leibesübungen* (Düsseldorf, 1927), 2 vols.

25. Georg Seiring, "Das Deutsche Hygiene-Museum in der Nachkriegszeit," *Hygienischer Wegweiser* 2 (1927): 27.

26. Martin Vogel, "Das Deutsche Hygiene-Museum Dresden," in *Grosse Ausstellung Düsseldorf 1926 für Gesundheitspflege, Soziale Fürsorge und Leibesübungen. Amtlicher Katalog* (Düsseldorf, 1926), p. 66.

27. Ibid., p. 65.

28. Later, of course, while eugenics movements in Britain and the USA promoted voluntary or compulsory sterilisation, race hygiene would be used to justify the mass murder of the Nazi holocaust. See Daniel Kevles, *In the Name of Eugenics: Genetics and the Uses of Human Heredity* (New York, 1985); *Darwin und Darwinismus: Eine Ausstellung zur Kultur- und Naturgeschichte* (Berlin, 1994).

29. Karl A. Lingner, *Der Mensch als Organisationsvorbild,* guest lecture given December 14, 1912 before the professoriate of the University of Bern (Bern, 1914).

30. *Das National-Hygiene-Museum* (n. 22 above), p. 6. Particularly impressive was a similar presentation technique – the "frost-cut" or "cryosection" technique – which was demonstrated, for example, at the "Anahyga," the German anatomical-hygienic exhibition entitled *Man*: "well-shaped male corpses, frozen and hardened, were cut into slices after a method of Prof. Rüdinger. The preparation is fixed on a stand and can be leafed through like

a book … Particularly interesting for the lay person is the sagittal median cut in the middle of the body, reaching almost all organs which are then represented in the intersection." *Illustrierte Führer durch die Anahyga, deutsche anatome. hygien. Ausstellung "Der Mensch"* (Munich, 1929), p. 28 ff.

31. Cellon, also called Cellhorn, a translucent synthetic plastic made by the Röhm & Haas A. G. Company, Darmstadt, subsequent supplier Dynamit-Aktiengesellschaft, formerly Alfred Nobel & Co., Troisdorf. Cellon is a celluloid-like substance derived from acetylcellulose but it is less easily combustible than celluloid. It can be worked mechanically and can also be glued. It has the disadvantages of turning yellow over long periods and the tendency to shrink with ageing of the material.

32. *Das National-Hygiene-Museum* (n. 22 above), p. 12.

33. Typed report by Isolde Seyfarth, née Ringelhahn, September 20, 1972 and July 7, 1993, Deutsches Hygiene-Museum, Archiv, Nr. 73/46.

34. Ibid.

35. Ibid.

36. Protokoll Vorstandssitzung DHM e.V. vom 24.6.1927, Deutsches Hygiene-Museum, Archiv, Nr. 18/6. Remarkably, this new development has not been protected by a patent. Relevant searches by the competent authorities remain fruitless.

37. Quoted from Bruno Gebhard, "Im Strom und Gegenstrom. 1919–1937," *Beiträge zur Geschichte der Wissenschaft und der Technik* 14 (1976): 4.

38. Konrad Wünsche, "Das Bildnis des durchsichtigen Gesunden oder: Die Wahrhaftigkeit des Gläsernen Menschen," in Beier and Roth, eds. (n. 2 above), p. 85 ff.

39. After Roth in Beier and Roth, eds. (n. 2 above), p. 41.

40. Gebhard (n. 37 above), p. 79.

41. Gebhard (n. 37 above), p. 46 and p. 68 ff.

42. "The Camp Transparent Woman," *The Corsetry and Underware Journal* (October 1936): 17.

43. Hermann Hebestreit and Robert Koenig, *Die Gläserne Fabrik. Ein Beitrag zur Gesundheits-führung in den Betrieben* (Dresden, 1938), p. 2.

44. *Report of the Scientific Management of the German Hygiene Museum: Central Institute for Hygienic Education*, 25 (1946), Deutsches Hygiene-Museum, Archiv, Nr. 46/36.

45. Deutsches Hygiene-Museum, Archiv, Nr. 40/37.

46. George Seiring, 1883–1972; first meeting with Lingner in 1906; Government Adviser before 1927; 1927, Honorary Doctor of Medicine of the Medical Faculty of Leipzig University; May 16, 1930, Honorary Senator/Councillor of the Dresden Technical College and President of the German Hygiene Museum; 1930/31, Managing Director and Vice-President of the International Hygiene Exhibition; moved to Cologne–Rheinfelden in 1947.

47. *Kölnische Rundschau*, July 28, 1950, and *Rheinische Zeitung*, July 28, 1950.

48. Not until 1955 was there once again a new Transparent Man from Dresden in West Germany, exhibited in Munich at the International Exhibition for Nutrition and Home Decor. Director Kunkel, back from Munich, reported in the *Sächsische Zeitung*, November 9, 1955, "If we explained to the visitors that our government spends over 30% of the budget for the health service, they would immediately compare this to the spending of the Bonn government. It became quickly obvious where the future of Germany lies."

49. *Sächsisches Tageblatt*, September 7, 1950.

50. H. Kern, who fitted the transparent figures, was able to experience Stalin's birthday celebrations. His impressions of the celebrations were reported in a somewhat unconsciously ambiguous way: "The climax of the experience was for Kern the moment when he saw Stalin for the first time and was moved by the effect of this strange man … this emotion almost gave him a feeling of tightness in his chest." From *Ein Dresdner sieht Moskau* (n.d., n.p.).

51. Staatsarchiv Dresden: Landesregierung Sachsen, Ministerpräsident, Nr. 1650, p. 131 ff.

52. Response of the German Hygiene Museum, dated August 19, 1961, Deutsches Hygiene-Museum, Archiv, Nr. 61/22.

53. Letter from the Minister of Employment and Health Affairs of the German Democratic Republic dated June 2, 1950, Deutsches Hygiene-Museum, Archiv, Nr. 50/15: "It is a fact that great interest also exists in the field of veterinary medicine for such teaching material. These transparent animals would also represent an important article in our export trade."

54. Modernisation of the Transparent Men had been the subject of much thought even before the German Hygiene Museum came under new management after the collapse of East

Germany and the fall of the Berlin Wall. **Very practical plans still survive from the years**. The intention was always to complement the static character of the figures by other media; however, not only a lack of finance, but also a fear that some feature of the attractiveness of the current presentation may be irretrievably lost, have so far left plans for change in abeyance.

55. Jörg Blech, "Bilderwut auf Krankenschein," *Die Zeit*, December 6, 1996.
56. Voxel-Man: ⟨⟨http://www.uke.uni-hamburg.de/Institutes/IMDM/IDV/VOXEL-MAN.html⟩⟩ and the Visible Human Project: ⟨⟨http://www.nlm.nih.gov/research/visible/visible_human.html⟩⟩.
57. Vesalius: ⟨⟨http://vesalius.com⟩⟩.

Ghislaine Lawrence

Design solutions for medical technology: Charles Drew's profound hypothermia apparatus for cardiac surgery

The modern medical specialty of open-heart surgery had its origins in the 1950s. The development of apparatus to take over the function of the patient's heart and lungs during surgery played a central role, and much of the early work was done in US medical centres. John Gibbon of Philadelphia was the first to operate successfully using a heart–lung machine, in 1953.[1] The Mayo Clinic subsequently modified Gibbon's machine for their own open-heart programme. At Minnesota University during 1954–55, C. Walton Lillehei championed his cross-circulation technique, in which a patient's relative took the place of a heart–lung machine. Lillehei later devised and used a heart–lung machine in collaboration with Richard DeWall.[2]

By 1960, these and other surgeons had established, if not standard procedures, then at least the feasibility of open-heart surgery using cardiopulmonary bypass and, potentially curative of otherwise fatal conditions such as congenital heart defects in children, open-heart surgery slowly came into routine use. In London, several teaching hospitals began programmes in the late 1950s or early 1960s. The adoption of new technology was an integral part of open-heart surgery in the early years and, in Britain, major decisions over heart–lung machines preoccupied many surgeons: should an expensive purchase be made from the USA, or should a "home-made" version be devised in the hospital workshops? Or indeed, as will be presented in this case study, should an altogether alternative form of technology be pursued?

***

The raison d'être of museums is, of course, their artefacts, and the "black boxes" of modern technology cause curators much angst, offering, at first sight, rather less potential for analysis than their more ornate and less opaque precursors. However, recent work in the history and sociology of technology offers much potential for the analysis and display of these modern artefacts. In this paper, both contingent factors and the specific culture of British operative surgery during a transitional period will be shown to have played key roles in deciding why a piece of surgical technology finally took the form it did.

***

Charles Drew's apparatus for his technique of open-heart surgery under profound hypothermia was developed around about 1960. The apparatus has been in the Science Museum's collections since 1987, and it went on permanent display in the *Health Matters* gallery in 1994. One of the principal intentions in that gallery was to make the selection of objects for display, and the display treatment itself, more in line with new perspectives in the history of medicine and of technology. With these concerns uppermost, it appeared to be a promising case study. There were, for example, extensive accounts of the design process, with striking evidence of industrial involvement and transfer of skills and technology from outside medicine. At an early stage, there had been much "ad hocery" and improvisation in the apparatus used. After initial acclaim, the technique had apparently been abandoned within a few years by most surgeons, but was still advocated by its inventor, so there was the promise of controversy. Subsequently, the method had been assessed as "not mainstream" – that is, not on the rather direct path that some historians maintain can be traced for the "development" of open-heart surgery.[3]

The major design work on Drew's apparatus was carried out between 1959 and 1961 at the Westminster Hospital, London, where Charles Drew (1916–87) was a thoracic surgeon.[4] By his own account, he was seeking a simpler way of doing open-heart surgery than using a heart–lung machine. In particular, it frustrated him that, when using a heart–lung machine, "the perfect oxygenator" (that is, the patient's own lungs) "lay fallow in the chest."[5] Heart–lung machines were, of course, designed to pump and oxygenate the patient's blood outside the body, thus bypassing both heart and lungs. Surgeons reported several problems with the models then available. Most of these were still unique "one-off" versions, devised by individual medical men in collaboration either with companies, such as IBM, General Motors or AGA, or with hospital physicists or engineering departments.[6]

The problems that surgeons in the 1950s most frequently associated with heart–lung machines were first, that they required large priming volumes of stored blood (which was detrimental to the patient's body chemistry and clotting functions) and second, that the artificial-lung component damaged the blood cells as they passed through it. However, less specific criticisms make it clear that, to many surgeons in the mid 1950s, heart–lung machines seemed just "complicated," and "difficult to run."[7]

Drew himself had tried a Lillehei–DeWall type heart–lung machine in 1955–56, during which period he experienced "difficulties, disappointments and the set-backs well known to everyone who has undertaken this type of work."[8]

Seeking an alternative to the use of a heart–lung machine, Drew developed the technique he called "profound hypothermia."[9] This involved cooling the patient down to about 15°C, at which point the heart stopped beating and the patient was, to all intents and purposes, clinically dead. Heart surgery could then be performed (with a self-imposed one-hour time limit) and the patient rewarmed, whereupon the heart usually restarted, either spontaneously or with electrical stimulation. In this way, Drew obviated the need for artificial oxygenation of the blood – this took place in the patient's own lungs, which could be artificially ventilated until, at low temperatures, they were not required. Since the 1930s, hypothermia had been the subject of considerable research, first as a potential cancer therapy, and then in relation to the survival of shipwrecks in the Second World War. Findings suggested that, in controlled cooling to low temperatures, the brain and heart might survive undamaged for limited periods with little or no oxygen.[10]

Drew did, of course, need the "pump" component of heart–lung machines for two purposes. First, he needed to be able to maintain the circulation of the blood artificially, in case the heart stopped during the cooling process but before sufficiently low temperatures had been reached (the usual cause of death in accidental exposure to cold). Second, in order to reach such low temperatures, he cooled the patient, not directly, but by cooling their blood in a heat exchanger as it circulated outside the body and then pumping the cooled blood back into them. In early case series, Drew's team used a makeshift heat exchanger for the blood that comprised steel tubes placed in a length of roof guttering, through which ran hot or cold water.[11] Subsequently, the much more sophisticated apparatus that is the subject of this paper was devised. It incorporated two "roller" blood pumps of a type used widely in extracorporeal bypass, but with an innovative annular heat exchanger mounted on trunnions and supplied with iced and hot water from a separate unit.

In the early 1960s, Drew's success rates with this apparatus were comparable to those of any of the small number of other surgeons doing open-heart work. (The patients were often children, open-heart surgery at that period being dominated by the repair of simple or moderately complex congenital heart defects sometimes known as "holes in the heart." Problems with the valves of the heart, such as those arising as long-term sequelae of rheumatic fever, were considered to be technically much more difficult.) In particular, Drew's success rates in correcting Fallot's tetralogy, a complex fourfold congenital abnormality, were better than those of other surgeons, with a mortality rate of 15%.[12]

However, if this apparatus was an initial success for Drew, in other ways it was a failure. It seems probable that only three more machines of this kind were ever produced, one for the other London hospital at which Drew performed open-heart surgery, St George's.[13] By the late 1960s, the only hospitals using profound hypothermia were the two at which Drew himself operated (the Westminster and St George's). An isolated "objective clinical trial" of the method, reviewing results at Bristol Royal Infirmary from 1960 to 1967, was published in 1968.[14]

Participants in heart surgery at that time recalled some apparently obvious and fairly unanimous reasons for the the demise of the technique.[15] First, it was said that the one-hour operating time limit grew increasingly irksome: as the repair of more complex defects involving the heart valves began to be attempted, even the faster surgeons found that one hour was not long enough to complete the operative repair; and second, it was recalled that the performance of heart–lung machines improved considerably during the 1960s. When asked why Drew persisted in using the technique of profound hypothermia for the rest of his career, to the extent that, by the mid 1970s, physicians were reluctant to refer patients to him for heart surgery because of it, several of those interviewed considered that the reason was simply that he had invented the technique, and was therefore wedded to it.

***

An *idée fixe* is perhaps one of the least appealing explanations for sociologically minded historians. Furthermore, the reasons for abandoning profound hypothermia given by cardiac surgeons – admittedly through the "retrospectoscope" – seemed so convincing. Could it be that this artefact, which had seemed so promising a candidate from the perspective of what might be called the "new" history of technology, was in fact an "open-and-shut" case? It seemed that some "problematisation" of the issues involved might prove fruitful. A number of other questions could be pursued, in particular those raised by the form of the apparatus itself, which might further illuminate issues to do with the success of the technique, the machine, or both. Why was it built as it was? Why did it look as it did? Drew's apparatus actually looked very *unlike* other medical equipment devised at this time (*see* Figure 1). The notion that form follows function has come under attack by historians of technology in recent years.[16] Might this machine have been built differently, looked different? First of all, did it have to be so big? It was very big – huge, given the size of the average operating theatre.

The design process is relatively well documented. It did not, as one might have expected at that time, involve a hospital physics or engineering department. The Westminster, Drew's own hospital, had a particularly active and innovative medical scientist in Percy Cliffe, who was well known for devising new apparatus and became head of the Department of Clinical Measurement there in 1959.[17] However Drew had it seems temporarily fallen out with Cliffe.[18] When he first began to think seriously of how to cool down his patients, Drew went, not to Cliffe, but to a copy of a standard engineering textbook – *An Introduction to Heat Transfer* by Fishenden and Saunders.[19] Finding it difficult reading, he consulted the senior author, Owen Saunders, then Professor of Mechanical Engineering at Imperial College, London.[20] Saunders put Drew in touch with a refrigeration engineer from the APV Company whom he had supervised for a Master's thesis on the cooling of non-Newtonian fluids. This led to an extremely close collaboration with the engineer in question, David Shore, and with APV, process engineers to the food industry working especially with brewing, and dairy and ice-cream plants.[21]

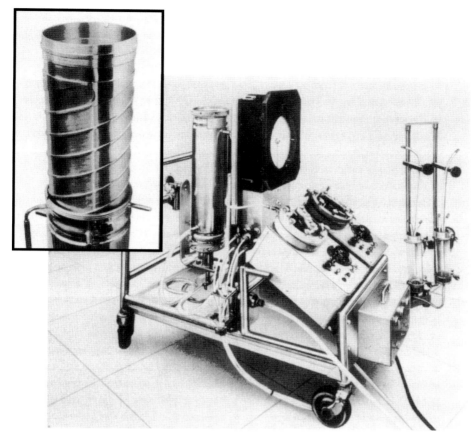

Figure 1 (left). The heat exchanger, blood pumps and control unit of the profound hypothermia apparatus designed for Charles Drew by the APV Company. The inset shows the internal construction of the heat exchanger.

Figure 2 (right). The heating and cooling unit of APV designed apparatus, which was sometimes placed outside the operating theatre.

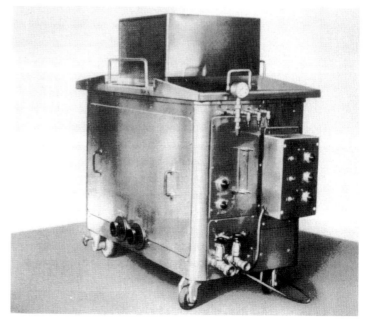

Shore eventually published full accounts of the design of the machine in a paper to the Institution of Mechanical Engineers and in the *Journal of Refrigeration*.[22] Both papers make reference to the choice of controls used on the apparatus. In the *Journal of Refrigeration*, Shore wrote that "The visual aid offered by pneumatic control, together with its simplicity, was considered by our design team to outweigh other merits of the electric or electronic control systems."[23] In his paper to the Institution of Mechanical Engineers, he stated that pneumatic controls were considered "more reliable than electric or electronic equipment."[24]

Here was a clear indication of a choice being made concerning the form of the machine – and the first suggestion that it might have been made differently. Further inquiry into this issue of the controls leads one to speculate about the reasons given for the use of pneumatic controls. A reluctance to use electronic controls was apparently widespread amongst mechanical engineers at this period. For example, the guidance notes for sales representatives of the Cambridge Scientific Instrument Company in the 1950s stated: "this craze for the use of electronic circuits as applied to measuring and recording instruments is often ill-founded and may be pressed to disadvantage for the user ... electronics is a great and potent means of furthering instrumentation ... use it if you must, but never if you need not."[25] Of course, Shore was not only a mechanical engineer but his company, APV, specialised in process engineering. Several authors have stressed how pneumatic controls were traditionally favoured in process control.[26] Their use goes some way towards explaining the size and general ungainliness of Drew's equipment: to operate the controls required air lines and a compressor, or an air bottle of 48 cubic feet capacity that would last for two operations.[27] An even larger component, however, was the heating and cooling unit for the supply of iced and hot water – so large that it was, in practice, usually accommodated outside the operating theatre, sometimes in a corridor or the anaesthetic room (*see* Figure 2). The design remit that Drew gave to Shore was to devise a heat exchanger capable of cooling a body weighing 150 pounds from 37°C to a mean of 15°C in half an hour, with an extracorporeal blood flow of 3 litres per minute, the blood temperature never rising above 40°C nor falling below 4°C.[28] Shore worked meticulously to these and other specifications, ever aware of the need for the apparatus to "fail to safety," and that he had a patient's life to consider, rather than the workings of an ice-cream plant. He devised an extremely sensitive annular form of heat exchanger. To secure precise control of the temperature of the water supplied to it, he provided a refrigeration unit with ice bank and heating element, and a safety valve that ensured the water simply recirculated in the event of a fault in the thermoregulation. This added considerably to the bulk and complexity of the equipment.

***

Having thus begun to consider how this apparatus might have been built differently, it seems logical to determine what apparatus was used by other teams practising profound hypothermia. It seems clear that the success of Drew's apparatus is a question rather separate from the success of the technique of profound hypothermia itself. Several leading cardiac centres *did* use profound hypothermia, with enthusiasm and with good success rates, for a period of about five years, when it was seen as a genuine alternative to heart–lung machines and thought to have considerable potential for the future.[29] It was the method of choice, for example, at St Bartholomew's Hospital from 1961 to 1965.[30] Clearly, the technique of profound hypothermia had a separate life from the apparatus designed by APV. What then, were the other teams using?

In London, at St Bartholomew's and also at King's College Hospital, open-heart surgery under profound hypothermia was performed with a piece of equipment devised within 18 months of Drew's, but in quite striking contrast to it.[31] Smaller and much less cumbersome, it was made by a company called New Electronic Products (NEP); not surprisingly, therefore, it had electronic controls. Other features resulted in a reduction

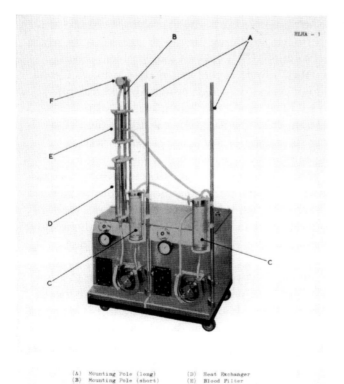

Figure 3. NEP apparatus used for profound hypothermia at St Bartholomew's Hospital, from the technical manual.

(A) Mounting Pole (long)   (D) Heat Exchanger
(B) Mounting Pole (short)   (E) Blood Filter
(C) Blood Reservoir   (F) Pressure Guage

APPARATUS SET UP FOR HYPOTHERMIA PERFUSION   Fig.16

in overall size. The heat exchanger was much smaller and simpler, and merely clamped to a pole, whereas in the APV machine the heat exchanger was mounted on trunnions so that it could be up-ended to allow air to escape. There was a separate refrigeration and heating unit, but this did not incorporate an ice bank, so was smaller than that with the APV machine; however, some surgeons did not go to the trouble of using it, preferring instead the water supply from an ordinary sink, and some ice.[32]

***

In many ways, the whole ethos of these two machines, designed for the same purpose within 18 months of each other, was entirely different. The machine that Shore designed at APV is redolent of his background in refrigeration and process engineering. It was large: space was rarely a problem in processing industries. The control element was immensely precise. In other details, instrumentation familiar to process control was chosen – the Taylor Fullscope recorder controller, for example, on which continuous circular records of inflow and outflow water temperature were plotted. This was unknown in medical instrumentation of the period. The NEP machine had a simple dial indicator instead.

The design problem was presented in a way that was very familiar to APV – an individual customer presenting them with a problem for which they designed a one-off solution. (APV had a strong problem-solving tradition: in later years, they solved the problem of the Cadbury's Creme Egg.[33]) What APV did not design were mass produced products; NEP, however, explicitly did so. They were a small company, founded in 1947. Some of their business came from the Royal Aircraft Establishment at Farnborough, for whom they designed miniature galvanometers; physiological recording equipment in general was an important part of their output.[34] Their "ethos," judging from surviving advertising material, was one of size reduction, self-containment and modular construction, all based on electronics.[35] Seen through half-closed eyes, as it were, their apparatus looks more "modern" than that of APV, perhaps partly because of its cream-painted sheet cladding. APV's use of stainless-steel and bent-tube construction gave their machine a similarity, not only to the dairy and brewing equipment they were used to producing, but to a style of hospital furniture that had been predominant since the years between the First and Second World Wars. Although there is no direct evidence of the involvement of industrial designers in the development of the NEP machine, it is noteworthy that their parent company, Honeywell, was one of the earliest to employ such specialists on a permanent basis.[36] One might speculate how much factors such as these, rather than those actually recalled by surgeons, influenced the limited success of the APV machine. As a study of the acquisition of computed tomography (CT) scanners by US radiologists in the 1970s has shown, the reasons that decision makers recall as underlying their acquisition of new technology – such as documented increased efficiency – frequently do not stand up to closer scrutiny.[37] Less often recalled reasons for acquisition may include, for example, institutional prestige, or the persuasive power of marketing techniques.

NEP marketed their machine themselves, but APV, once satisfied that their apparatus was working satisfactorily, passed this function to the company Allen & Hanburys, apparently considering that it was too far from their normal line of business to undertake the marketing effectively themselves.[38] The choice was perhaps not fortuitous. Allen & Hanburys were an old-established firm, founded in 1715, who made proprietary medicines, surgical instruments and hospital furniture;[39] they had no tradition of making or selling scientific instruments. Comparison of their advertising material with that of NEP is interesting. In the brochure that Allen & Hanburys produced to promote the APV apparatus, the front cover is devoted to a large, architectural photograph of the Westminster Hospital. The imposing nature of the building is accentuated by the low camera angle, invoking all the connotations of tradition and authority associated with a London teaching hospital (*see* Figure 4). NEP's advertising looked quite different. Promotional material for their profound hypothermia apparatus has not been traced, but leaflets produced to advertise other pieces of medical equipment at the same period have been preserved (*see* Figure 5).[40] They feature brightly coloured, "contemporary" artwork, rather than black-and-white photography; the stylised image of a hand brings connotations of ease of use and compactness; the company's affiliation to Honeywell Controls, suppliers of instrumentation to the US space programme, is prominently mentioned. In contrast, Allen & Hanburys chose to emphasise their product's association with an old and venerated medical institution. By deciding to call it the "Westminster Profound Hypothermia Apparatus" they had almost, if not quite, reverted to a tradition predominant in the medical supply trade throughout the nineteenth and early twentieth centuries – that of eponymous naming. They did not go so far as to call it the "Drew apparatus," but they did the next best thing, naming it after his *alma mater*. This tradition was dying elsewhere in the rapidly expanding field of medical equipment. It is perhaps not difficult to see how to some the NEP machine, with its connotations of scientific precision, greater air of "modernity," small size and possibly industrially designed shape, might have proved more attractive than APV's larger machine which was marketed on authority and tradition.

These contrasts in advertising practice, and in the two machines themselves, can, I believe, be linked to considerable change in surgical practice after the Second World War. In the rhetoric of the newer surgical specialties of the 1950s and 1960s, there are some words that occur repeatedly. One is the word "new" itself, and another is the word "scientific;" but there is a third word – "teamwork" – which it is interesting

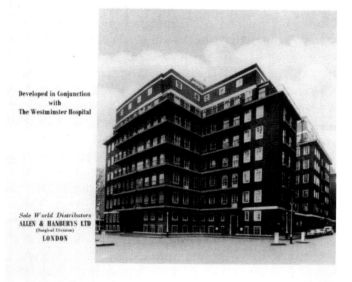

The **Westminster** PROFOUND HYPOTHERMIA UNIT

Developed in Conjunction
with
The Westminster Hospital

Sole World Distributors
ALLEN & HANBURYS LTD
(Surgical Division)
LONDON

*Figure 4. Front cover of Allen & Hanburys
advertising brochure for Drew's profound
hypothermia apparatus, showing the
Westminster Hospital.*

to explore in relation to Drew's apparatus. Nowhere was use of this word more prominent than in the area of open-heart surgery. In this emergent specialty, existing groups, such as anaesthetists, took on far more central roles. New groups came into being, especially of paramedics occupying key positions, for example as pump technicians. New degrees of liaison and interdependency were set up, not only inside the operating theatre, but outside it too – in postoperative intensive care, for example – and with cardiac physicians, on whom surgeons were dependent for the preoperative assessment of patients and, indeed, for referring patients to them in the first place. As one leading heart surgeon of the period recalled, surgeons had to make the transition from being "captain of the ship" to being "chairman of the board."[41] Not all of them made it; it seems possible that Charles Drew himself failed to make it. He was recalled by many as autocratic in theatre. He did not hesitate to curse his junior staff, but was quick to make amends, and inspired fierce loyalty: one doctor who had worked for him as a house surgeon referred to himself as being one of a group known as "Drew's boys," and recalled how some of them would pretend not to hear the consultant anaesthetist's interjections during an operation, taking notice only of Drew himself – hardly a situation conducive to team-building.[42] It seems very likely that Drew was a captain of the ship and not a chairman of the board. In view of this, it is perhaps not surprising that he devised his machine largely independently of colleagues in other medical specialties – specialties that were to become essential to successful open-heart surgery. As mentioned above, he bypassed Percy Cliffe, the inventive medical scientist at the Westminster, a "natural" for Drew's project if ever there was one, because he had apparently fallen out with him. Drew the surgeon worked with Shore the engineer to produce a machine that satisfied the surgeon's and the engineer's criteria. The technique of profound hypothermia itself, alone of any other used in open-heart surgery of the period or since, produced a still, bloodless heart – the perfect operating conditions for the surgeon. In engineering terms, Shore's heat exchanger was more sophisticated than any other used in open-heart surgery in Britain or abroad.[43]

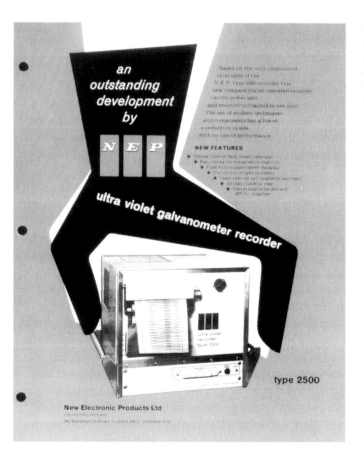

Figure 5. Example of NEP advertising literature from the early 1960s. The stylised image of a hand, in black on a bright red background, had a contemporary feel. It brought connotations of ease of use and compactness.

The concerns of other workers, however, were not always addressed. Two consultants referred, independently, their concerns over Drew's apparatus. One was an anaesthetist, who recalled that the low priming volume – a specific request of Drew's, to avoid the problems of stored blood meant that, if there were any obstruction in the blood circuits, the reservoirs would run dry in seconds, pumping air into the patient's circulation, with potentially fatal results.[44] This machine, which produced almost perfect operating conditions for the surgeon, required nerves of steel in the anaesthetist or pump technician who ran it. For other groups, such as the theatre staff who set up and dismantled it, taking several hours in all, the machine also had disadvantages.

It might not be impossible to write an account of these machines comparable to that produced by Pinch and Bijker for the bicycle – showing how the relative strengths of various interest groups affected the ultimate design.[45] In contrast to Drew's machine, the NEP apparatus was designed by a trio of consultant surgeon, anaesthetist and physiologist.[46] Several design features demonstrated concern for the various team members' jobs, not just the surgeon's. Photosensitive safety devices were fitted, for example, to give audible alarms if the reservoirs were in danger of running dry. A special feature was made of the fact that the machine operator could sit facing the operation, which apparently was not possible with Drew's machine. It was much simpler to assemble, take apart and sterilise. It probably cost less, too. It is possible that Allen & Hanburys might have sold the APV apparatus almost at cost, in order to launch a new product of this kind. Even so, the price was likely to have been more than £1000.[47] Charles Drew himself was largely freed from financial constraints in his research, by an endowment from a grateful and wealthy benefactor.[48]

***

It is possible to see the Westminster apparatus for profound hypothermia as an embodiment of Charles Drew's concerns and priorities and perhaps somewhat autocratic tendencies, his preferred ways of working, and the prevailing institutional and financial circumstances that allowed these a fairly free rein. Further evidence for this interpretation comes from the typescript of a lecture that Drew gave in Tokyo in 1968. His collaboration with David Shore and APV continued more or less throughout the 1960s, and by this time Drew had made several modifications to his original extracorporeal circuit, most notably in substituting a single reservoir for separate ones in the right and left circuits. By 1968, he was considering discarding reservoirs entirely, replacing them with heat exchangers, using a shunt between the two venous lines to equalize flow through the pumps, using the same shunt line for the giving of blood, and at the same time removing air from the lines to the heart immediately after cannulation. He had very particular reasons for doing this. "Such a circuit," Drew wrote, "could be placed at the head of the table and manipulated by the surgeon, for this reason: during cooling the surgeon is not concerned with the open heart and can therefore control the extracorporeal circulation; during open heart surgery, the extracorporeal circulation is no longer used. When he has finished his manipulations in the heart, he can resume control of the extracorporeal circulation."[49] Here, indeed, is clear evidence of Drew's wish to take responsibility for every aspect of open-heart surgery, rather than distribute functions among a team, and of how this might very literally be translated into the design of apparatus. Drew's former senior registrar, John Bailey, on being read this quote, exclaimed "Oh yes, it was one of Charles' greatest aims to get rid of the perfusionist!"[50]

This is yet more supporting evidence, it seems, for the claim by certain historians of technology that machines are not adequately described by a single overt function. Charles Drew's apparatus was intended to cool patients to very low temperatures, but, at least in later forms, it seems it was also intended, consciously or otherwise, to "get rid of the perfusionist." Likewise, success is not measured solely in terms of performance specifications. One retired woman cardiac surgeon recalled how much she liked profound hypothermia because it was "so neat and tidy."[51]

When it comes to form, of course, all engineering solutions are "borrowed," but looking at where from, and why, can provide surprising insights.

Notes

1. J. H. Gibbon, Jr, "Application of a Mechanical Heart and Lung Apparatus to Cardiac Surgery," in *Recent Advances in Cardiovascular Physiology and Surgery* (Minneapolis, 1953), pp. 107–13. For an account of Gibbon and his work, see A. Romaine-Davis, *John Gibbon and His Heart–Lung Machine* (Philadelphia, 1991).
2. C. W. Lillehei, R. L. Varco, M. Cohen et al., "The First Open Heart Repairs of Ventricular Septal Defect, Atrioventricular Communis, and Tetralogy of Fallot Using Extracorporeal Circulation by Cross-circulation: A Thirty Year Follow-up," *Annals of Thoracic Surgery* 41 (1986): 4–21.
3. See, for example, G. Clowes, Jr, "The Historical Development of the Surgical Treatment of Heart Disease," *Bulletin of the History of Medicine* 34 (1960): 29–51.
4. "Obituary, Mr Charles Drew," *The Times*, June 6, 1987.
5. Drew papers, undated typescript, Holme Lecture, given by Drew at University College Hospital Medical School, p. 2.
6. Gibbon, and later the Mayo Clinic, worked with IBM. General Motors built a heart–lung machine for F. D. Dodrill in Detroit. See Romaine-Davis (n. 1 above), p. 139.
7. D. C. Cooley, "Perspectives in Cardiac Surgery with Personal Reflections," *Surgical Clinics of North America* 58 (1978): 895–906.
8. C. E. Drew et al., "Experimental Approach to Visual Intracardiac Surgery, Using an Extracorporeal Circulation," *British Medical Journal* 2 (1957): 1323–29, and Drew (n. 5 above), p. 2.
9. C. E. Drew, G. Keen, and D. B. Benazon, "Profound Hypothermia," *The Lancet* 1 (1959): 745–47; C. E. Drew and I. M. Anderson, "Profound Hypothermia in Cardiac Surgery: Report of Three Cases," *The Lancet* 1 (1959): 748–50.
10. O. G. Edholm, "Hypothermia and the Effects of Cold: Introduction," *British Medical Bulletin* 17, no. 1 (1961): 1–4. The whole issue was devoted to this subject.

11. C. E. Drew, "Cardiac Surgery at the Westminster Hospital," *Broadway,* Westminster Medical School Journal (March 1966): 25–27.

12. For an analysis of Drew's results see T. B. Boulton and R. L. Hurt, "The Drew Technique of Profound Hypothermia for Cardiac Surgery in the 1960s," in *Technologies of Modern Medicine*, ed. G. M. Lawrence (London, 1994), pp. 25–39, 34.

13. A machine of this design was also in use at the Brook Hospital, London. It is possible that another was exported to France.

14. R. H. Belsey et al., "Profound Hypothermia in Cardiac Surgery," *Journal of Thoracic and Cardiovascular Surgery* 56, no. 4 (1968): 497–509.

15. Interview of J. Bailey by G. Lawrence, April 15, 1996; interview of M. Braimbridge by G. Lawrence, September 27, 1995; interview of M. Sturridge by G. Lawrence, November 2, 1995; interview of W. Williamson by G. Lawrence, July 12, 1995; and see Boulton and Hurt (n. 12 above), p. 36.

16. See, for example, S. Lubar, "Culture and Technological Design in the 19th Century Pin Industry: John Howe and the Howe Manufacturing Company," *Technology and Culture* 28 (1987): 253–82.

17. "Obituary, P. Cliffe," *British Medical Journal* 305 (1992): 1154.

18. Interview of W. Williamson (n. 15 above).

19. M. Fishenden and O. A. Saunders, *An Introduction to Heat Transfer* (Oxford, 1950).

20. Interview of D. Shore by G. Lawrence and T. Boon, July 13, 1993.

21. G. A. Dummett, *From Little Acorns: A History of the APV Company Ltd* (London, 1981).

22. D. T. Shore, "Heat Exchange in Profound Hypothermia: Heat Exchanger Design for Blood During External Circulation," *Proceedings of the Institution of Mechanical Engineers, Thermodynamics and Fluid Mechanics Group 9 Jan 1963* (1963); D. T. Shore, "Profound Hypothermia," *Journal of Refrigeration* (May/June 1961): 50–52.

23. Shore (n. 22 above), p. 51.

24. Ibid., p. 10.

25. Quoted in A. Anderson, "The Story of Cambridge Instruments," *New Scientist* 114 (June 11, 1987): 57–58, a review of M. J. G. Cattermole and A. F. Wolfe, *Horace Darwin's Shop: A History of the Cambridge Scientific Instrument Company, 1878–1968* (Bristol, 1987).

26. J. T. Stock, "Pneumatic Process Controllers: The Early History of Some Basic Components," *Transactions of the Newcomen Society* 56 (1984–85): 169–78.

27. Shore (n. 22 above), p. 11.

28. Ibid., p. 5.

29. D. G. Melrose wrote in 1961 that profound hypothermia was "inherently simple in equipment and sparing of blood ... a most interesting field and one which may alter our present concepts." D. G. Melrose, "Types of Heart–Lung Machines Used in Extra-Corporeal Circulation," *Postgraduate Medical Journal* 37 (1961): 639–45.

30. Boulton and Hurt (n. 12 above), p. 30. King's College and The Brook Hospitals also used the technique in the early 1960s.

31. R. L. Hurt, "Apparatus for Profound Hypothermia by the Drew Technique," *The Lancet* 1 (1962): 783.

32. Personal communication, R. Hurt, December 29, 1995.

33. Interview of Shore (n. 20 above). The problem was to keep the yellow "yolk" separate from the "white" in the fondant filling of the chocolate egg.

34. Interview of R. Schild by G. Lawrence, February 10, 1997.

35. NEP Ltd. Industrial catalogue 1961–62, Science Museum Library Trade Literature Collection.

36. G. Hart, "Design Management: An I. D. Service for Capital Goods," *Design* 187 (1964): 46–53.

37. S. R. Baker, "The Diffusion of High Technology Medical Innovation: The Computed Tomography Scanner Example," *Social Science and Medicine* 13, pt. D (1979): 155–62.

38. Interview of Shore (n. 20 above).

39. G. Tweedale, *At the Sign of the Plough: 275 Years of Allen & Hanburys and the British Pharmaceutical Industry, 1715–1990* (London, 1990). A merger with Glaxo took place in 1958, but "during the 1960s, Allen & Hanburys continued very much as an independent company," p. 195.

40. Trade Literature Collection, Science Museum Library.

41. Interview of M. Braimbridge (n. 15 above).
42. Interview of T. Gould by G. Lawrence, June 29, 1995.
43. I. W. Brown at Duke University devised a new blood heat exchanger for use with extracorporeal circulation with the Harrison Radiator Division of General Motors Corporation in 1958, although not for profound hypothermia. I. W. Brown et al., "An Efficient Blood Heat Exchanger for Use With Extracorporeal Circulation," *Surgery* 44 (1958): 372–77. It used the simpler multitube design, however, which Shore considered unsuitable. See Shore (n. 22 above), p. 7.
44. Interview of J. Gil-Rodriguez by G. Lawrence, January 18, 1996.
45. T. Pinch and W. Bijker, "The Social Construction of Facts and Artefacts: Or How the Sociology of Science and the Sociology of Technology Might Benefit Each Other," *Social Studies of Science* 14 (1984): 399–441.
46. R. L. Hurt, *The Lancet* 1 (1964): 1198.
47. Interview of R. Myer by G. Lawrence, May 24, 1996.
48. Interview of J. Bailey (n. 15 above).
49. Drew Papers, typescript, "P. H. Tokyo June '68," p. 17.
50. Interview of J. Bailey (n. 15 above).
51. Interview of B. Slesser by G. Lawrence, May 5, 1996.

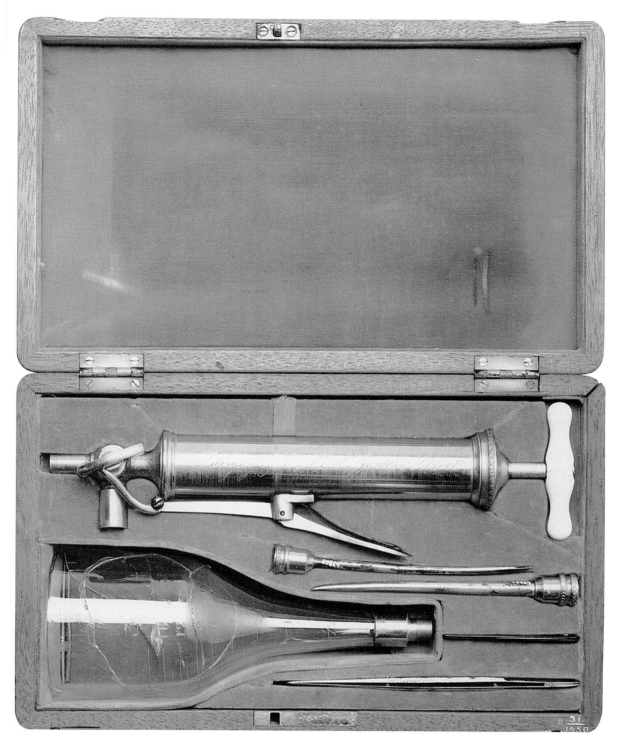

Syringe-based apparatus made in accordance with Blundell's specifications by Savigny, from the Wellcome Collections at the Science Museum (A 43853).

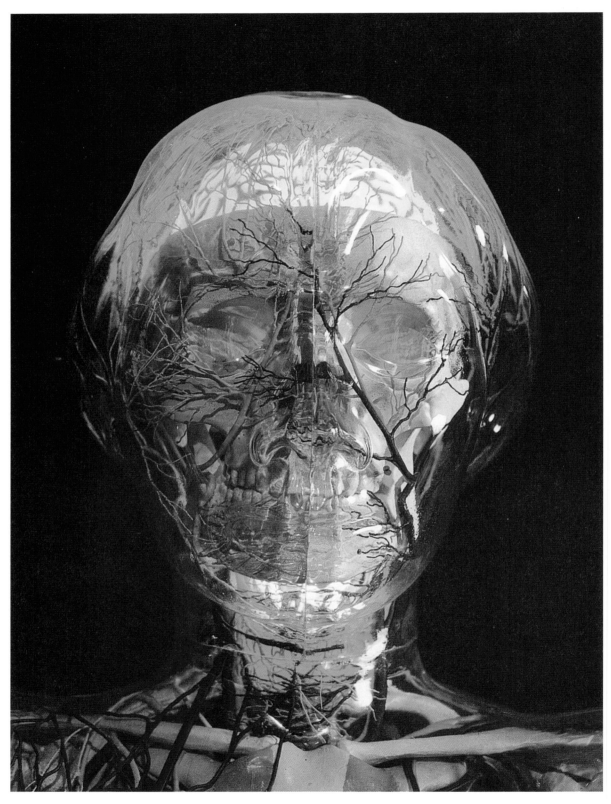

Detail of the head of the Transparent Woman on display in the German Hygiene Museum, 1998. Photograph Volker Kreidler.

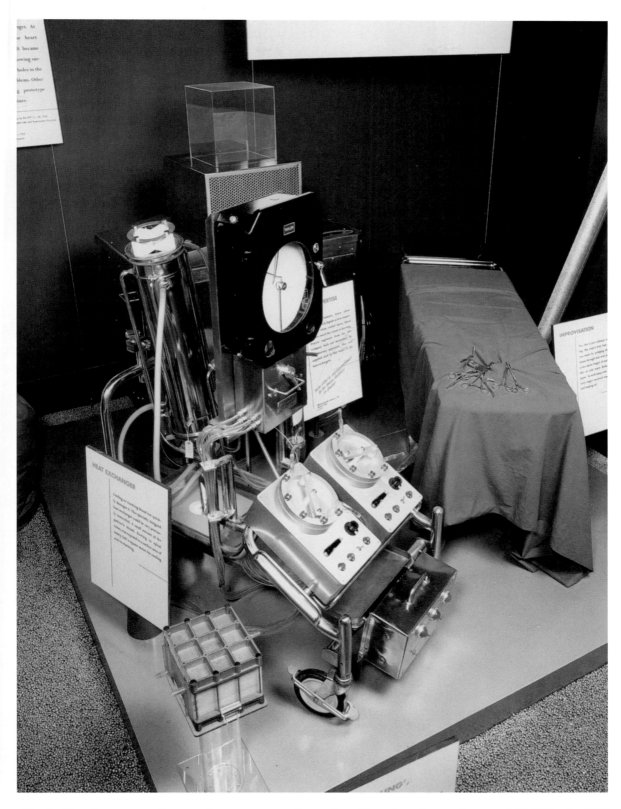

Charles Drew's apparatus for open-heart surgery under profound hypothermia, made around 1960 by the APV Company, in the Health Matters gallery, Science Museum, London. Science Museum inv. no 1985–410.

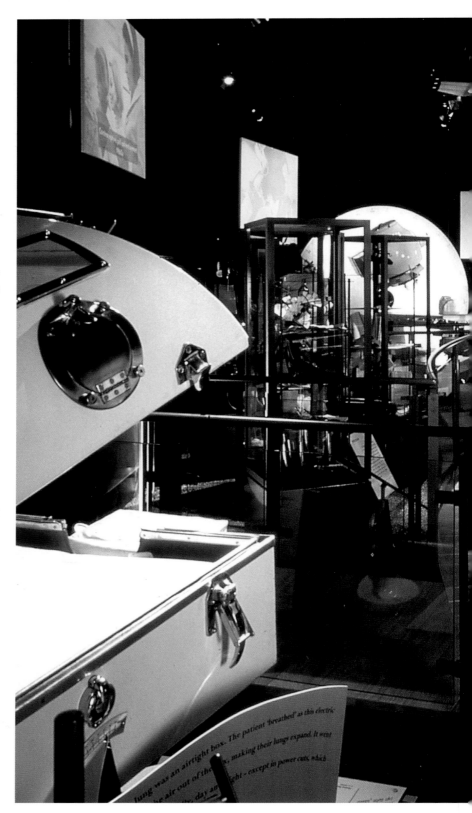

Section One of the Science Museum's Health Matters *gallery,* The Rise of Medicine.

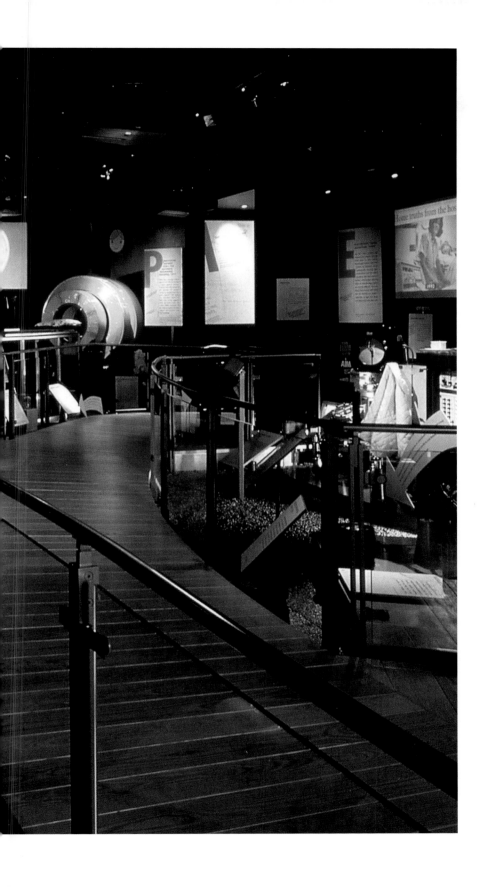

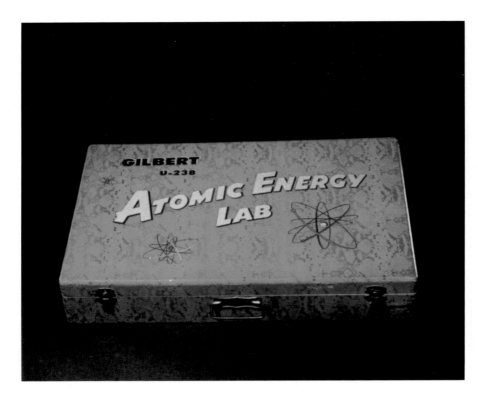

Gilbert U-238 Atomic Energy Lab by A.C. Gilbert Company (1950s).

The set contains a cloud chamber, Geiger-Müller counter, an electroscope and an electric eye kit. Such experimental kits with a Geiger counter were sold in the United States as well as in Germany. These devices made radiation measurements appear to be merely a trivial task. National Museum of American History (Catalog number 1990.0534).

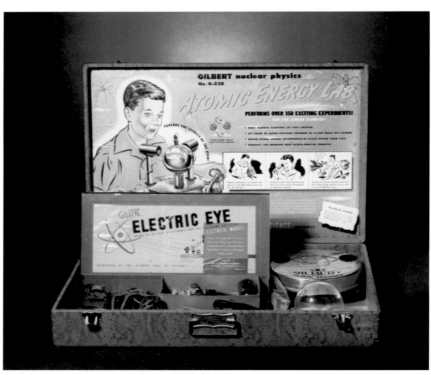

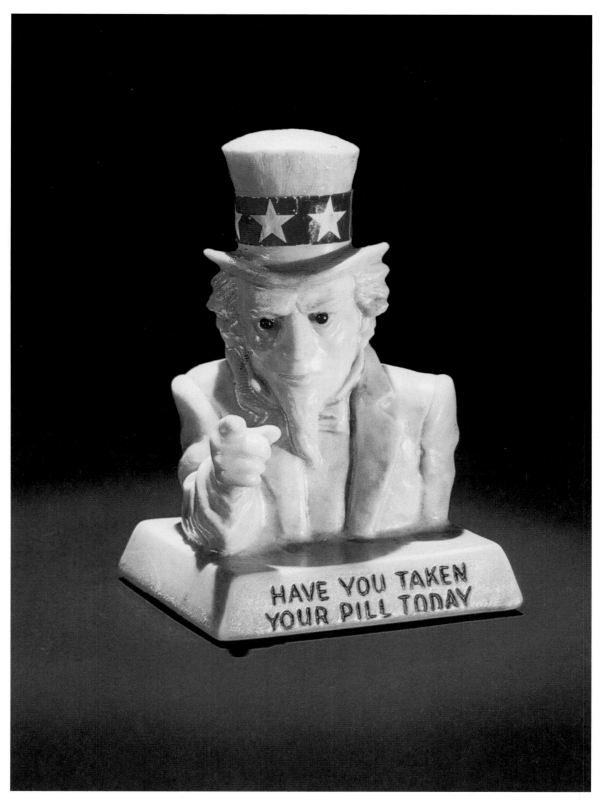

This Uncle Sam figurine asks "Have you taken your pill today?" It dates from 1969 protests over the distribution of oral contraceptives through US government-funded health clinics.

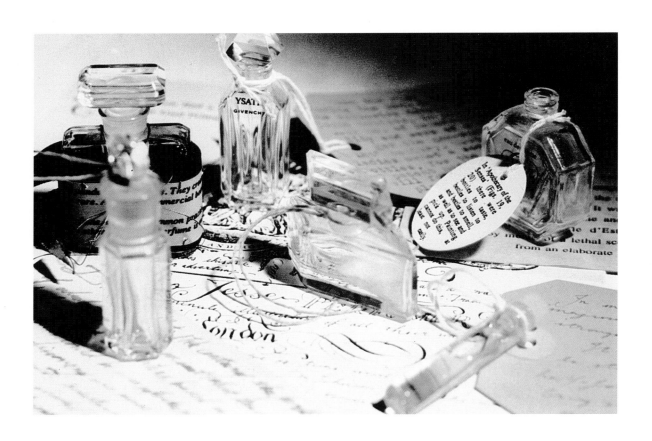

Pharmaceutical bottles by Mariko Jesse, 1995. In the Wellcome Trust exhibition Materia Medica *these artist-fabricated bottles were juxtaposed with historical examples.*

Johannes Abele

Safety clicks. The Geiger–Müller tube and radiation protection in Germany, 1928–1960

In 1956, the headline of a German newspaper read: "Are We Already Contaminated? Geiger Counters on Alpine Pastures."[1] The article described citizens enjoying themselves in the picturesque market place in Freiburg, drinking a glass of wine – which contained radioactive strontium: nuclear fallout had contaminated the environment and the food. The journalist then sought to calm the worries of the readers: "Death is not hiding in a glass of wine or a cup of milk."[2] In the face of day-to-day radiation hazards, it was necessary to re-assess the definition of safety, and in the course of this cultural development, radiation-measuring instruments gained particular importance. Although a range of different instruments such as ionisation chambers, photographic films or scintillation counters was used for radiation protection, for the general public it was the Geiger–Müller counter that symbolised the efforts to achieve radiation safety – it was even called the "watchdog of the atomic age."[3] For this reason, it is worth studying how that instrument's visible and audible representations of radioactivity achieved such significance.

The invention of the Geiger–Müller tube solved a challenging problem in science: the detection of particles and radiation that the human senses could not detect.[4] However, as this is a feature of all radiation-measuring instruments, it cannot sufficiently explain the Geiger counter's popularity. As an instrument that could make palpable radiations that fell beyond the ken of human senses, the Geiger counter came to represent health and safety in the face of unseen dangers. For both technical and socio-psychological reasons, the Geiger counter achieved a central role in the establishment and demonstration of safety measures. This paper relates the design of Geiger counters to distinct concepts for the preservation of public health and safety.

The focus of this study raises the more general question of how objects affect the creation of order in the social and cultural environment. Studies in material culture have pointed out the dialectical relationship between artefacts and social practice.[5] Accordingly, the design of Geiger–Müller counters resulted from scientists' reflections on radiation protection. Once produced, the instruments formed a powerful medium for structuring the practice of radiation protection: the devices defined *control procedures*, their material nature legitimised a *social order* related to radiation control, and the appearance of the instruments carried a *symbolic meaning* representing radiation safety.

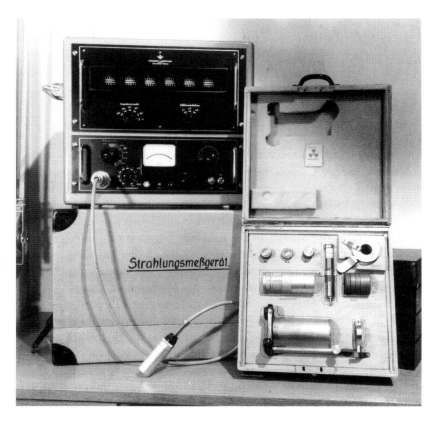

Figure 1. Exhibition of a Geiger–Müller counter at the Nuclear Research Centre Karlsruhe.

Why is the main emphasis of this study on concepts of radiation protection and not on their practical enforcement? Scientists and government officials involved in the organisation of radiation safety also discussed the design of measuring instruments. Their expertise crucially informed instrument manufacturing. The design of these instruments therefore expresses safety concepts that were not immediately linked to actual measuring practices.

In this paper, I will first briefly comment on the mode of operation of the Geiger–Müller tube and the history of nuclear research in Germany. The following paragraphs deal with the history of radiation-measuring instruments that have been constructed for a range of different atomic hazards: radiation exposure in the workplace,[6] nuclear fallout in the environment, and nuclear war. Variations in the design and use of measuring instruments reflected strategies to deal with different nuclear hazards that affected increasing sections of the population and involved supposedly less-qualified people in radiation measurements. Finally, I will reflect on the public debate about the so-called "Volks-Geiger counter," in which the instruments themselves became a representation of radiation safety.

The time span of this study is set by the invention of the Geiger–Müller tube in 1928, and the implementation of atomic legislation in the early 1960s. The post-war period deals only with radiation protection in West Germany.

The Geiger–Müller Counter

So far, I have spoken about the so-called Geiger counter as if it existed as a clearly defined object. However, the Geiger–Müller tube offers, rather, a generic *method* of counting. It is not a single specific *artefact*. According to its formal definition, the Geiger–Müller tube is merely a radiation detector working on a specific kind of gas amplification, with the possibility of a wide range of designs and types. Installations comprising such detectors, an amplifier and registration devices, have been colloquially called "Geiger counters" (Figure 1).

The Geiger–Müller tube converts ionising radiation into electric pulses. These pulses are then transformed by electronic amplifiers: pulse shaping, pulse generation and clipping are methods used to produce uniform pulses. The amplifiers thereby process the incoming information and generate clear and unambiguous signals. Finally, the configuration of the Geiger counter shapes the ways in which it is possible to perceive radiation: the clicks of a loudspeaker, the numbers on automatic counters, and also the movement of an indicator have become representations of radiation.

A wide range of instruments utilise the counting method of Geiger and Müller. These devices differ fundamentally in size and shape, materials, and function. By 1960, radiation-measuring instruments allowed a direct reading of the number of counts, indication of pulses per minute and of the dose rate, and measurement of different levels of radiation – all with only one instrument and the construction of optical and acoustic warning systems. Differences in the design of the instruments depended on various measurement factors. However, the appearance of these objects cannot be explained simply by reference to different functions; the different instrument designs also reflect different concepts of radiation control.

The Geiger–Müller Tube Before the Second World War

Many features of the Geiger–Müller tube used in the 1950s for radiation protection were developed in the 1930s. Hans Geiger and his research assistant, Walther Müller, invented the electrical method of counting radioactive particles that is now known as the "Geiger–Müller tube" in 1928. In contrast to the optical method of counting tiny flashes on a scintillation screen, electrical methods relied on the electrical effects of particles. Geiger's interest in the electrical counting of radiation dated from his early experiments in Ernest Rutherford's laboratory in Manchester in 1908. After his move to the radioactivity laboratory of the "Physikalisch-Technische Reichsanstalt" in Berlin in 1911, Geiger continued with further experiments on the measurement of individual particles which resulted in a new type of electrical detector, the Geiger point counter. In spite of an obvious lack of clarity about the reliability and practical utility of the counter, the detector came to be used in a number of significant experiments in the early 1920s. In 1925, Geiger left Berlin in order to become Professor of Physics at Kiel University. Müller was one of his first

PhD students there. He performed the experiments that finally led to the invention of the Geiger–Müller tube.[7]

It was the presumed sensitivity of the apparatus that caught the attention of the physics community. In their first publications, Geiger and Müller emphasised the capability of the tube to indicate even the weakest radiation. In comparing methods of measurement, "sensitivity" was defined in practice as the ability to measure a small amount of radiation in a short period of time. The practical time management of radiation investigations was a strong motivation for the use and further technical development of the Geiger–Müller tube.[8]

Geiger skilfully managed the presentation of the new apparatus. A number of physicists visited his laboratory in Kiel and observed the counter in action. Niels Bohr himself is said to have played around with it, as happy as a small child. Geiger and Müller also attended a number of conferences, where they demonstrated the working of the counting tube. Installing a loudspeaker, they impressed their colleagues with the clicks of the new apparatus. They conveyed the sensation of an immediate perception of radiation accessible hitherto only by the means of complex and lengthy experiments.[9] The Geiger–Müller tube thus became an instrument, not only for the *measurement* of radiation, but also for *public demonstration*, even though that was, as yet, to a very select audience.

Jeff Hughes has shown that the further practical development of the Geiger–Müller counter was crucially linked to the emerging "wireless" (radio) industry of the 1920s. These links transformed the practice and organisation of atomic physics, the techniques of which had been called into question in the course of serious controversies about the certainty of radioactivity measurements. Electronic amplifiers made the use of loudspeakers and mechanical counters possible. The new electronic technologies allowed the *automatic* registration of radiation, and thereby reduced the active involvement of physicists, who had previously been essential in the process of measurement. The automatic counting of ionising particles became common practice in scientific laboratories – although it remained a delicate task to overcome practical difficulties in the construction and operation of the counting devices.[10]

In the 1930s, the instrument proved useful in investigations of cosmic rays, neutron physics and work related to the German "uranium machine." Instruments and common experimental practices had been crucial to the emergence of a nuclear physics community.[11] However, the uses of the Geiger–Müller tube were not confined to the boundaries of physics laboratories. Since 1934, Boris Rajewsky had been examining several cases of human contamination in the radium industry; he was Director of the Institute of the Physical Foundations of Medicine at Frankfurt University.[12] In 1937, his institute became the "Kaiser-Wilhelm-Institut" of Biophysics, where Rajewsky established a centre for the investigation of radiation injuries. The ability to measure radiation in the human body was crucial for the diagnosis and therapy of "radium poisoning" or "radium infection" – the contemporary terms for the intake of radioactive elements, and the Geiger–Müller tube became a predominant device in Rajewsky's investigations. He was seriously concerned by the duration of existing medical examinations, in which weakened patients were exposed to time-consuming measurements of small quantities of radioactive substances deposited in their bodies. Because of the sensitivity of the counting tube, he hoped to be able to reduce the time required for the measurements.[13]

The transfer of the Geiger–Müller tube from physics laboratories to medical centres required changes in the operation of the instrument. The design of the control panel and the registration of the signals were adjusted for the convenience of the physicians, as they were unfamiliar with the technicalities of the instrument. In order to introduce the Geiger–Müller counter into medical practice, Rajewsky even drew an analogy to one of the most common medical instruments – he called the detector, fixed to a flexible tube, a "radiation stethoscope." Like the stethoscope, it allowed an examination of the organs and the diagnosis of localised physical defects.[14] Whereas other ways of measuring radiation in the human body indicated only whole-body activity, the Geiger–Müller tube allowed local measurement of radioactivity.[15] Rajewsky used the Geiger–Müller tube not only for medical examinations, but also in the search for uranium ores. In the early 1940s, he developed these instruments on the basis of previous applications in geological fieldwork.[16]

In the late 1930s, the first German *commercial* Geiger counters entered the market. These were designed for radiation protection in hospitals. Radium tubes were frequently lost or misplaced in hospitals, not only leading to economic losses, but also posing a danger to the health of patients and employees. Geiger–Müller tubes could find lost radium. The commercial counters were easily portable, being equipped with a battery or mains connection and stored in a box. Whereas physicists working in laboratories had struggled to achieve quantitative interpretations of their data, the commercial instruments offered impressive ways of representing detections: clicking loudspeakers, mechanical counters and flashing lights. If we can believe the advertisements, one had only to flick a switch – and the counter was ready for use.[17]

By the end of the Second World War, Geiger counters had been used for physical research, medical examinations and also for radiation measurements in buildings and in the environment. In the 1950s, these implementations were linked, in order to guarantee radiation safety.

Nuclear Research and Industries in Post-War Germany
After the Second World War, German physicists were occupied with the re-organisation of scientific research and teaching. Struggling with the material devastations of the War, at the same time they also attempted to overcome the intellectual isolation that had resulted from the National-Socialist regime. In the course of "Operation Paperclip," physicists worked

in the USA and thereby became familiar with what they saw as the enormous advancements of American science.[18] The encounters of German physicists with post-war nuclear physics in the USA and Great Britain left a deep impression; they met a level of scientific co-operation and of government involvement that was not yet known at home. The feeling that Germany had fallen behind in the field of atomic research and industries constituted a continuing justification for further research and industrial development in Germany.[19] The development of measuring instruments, the enforcement of safety regulations and the handling of public relations relied on examples from the USA, France and Britain.

Until 1955, atomic research in Germany was restricted by Allied control. The construction of nuclear reactors, isotope separation plants and large accelerators was forbidden. However, from 1948, Britain's Atomic Energy Research Establishment delivered isotopes to the Federal Republic of Germany for medical applications and non-military research. In addition, public funding provided by the Ministry of the Interior for civil defence supported nuclear research. This allowed circumvention of some legal restrictions. Allied control of nuclear research ended when the Federal Republic of Germany gained sovereignty in 1955; the Ministry of Atomic Energy co-ordinated efforts in the new field of scientific and industrial development. In the following years, the nuclear industries grew rapidly. The Federal Government and the states established three nuclear research centres in Karlsruhe, Jülich and Geesthacht near Hamburg. Universities in Munich, Frankfurt and Berlin built research reactors. The first nuclear power station near Kahl went into operation in 1961.[20]

The euphoric belief in atomic energy brought radioactivity into the centre of politics. The political and economic significance ascribed to nuclear research and industry dramatically changed the public role of atomic scientists. They increasingly moved from the laboratory bench to the conference table in Bonn. Nuclear scientists of the pre-war period became members of government advisory commissions.[21] Many former colleagues of Hans Geiger and their students crucially influenced regulatory policies. Their expertise in the measuring technologies for physical, medical and geological investigations became relevant to the problem of radiation protection. Instruments and practices that had been developed in the context of physical or medical research in the 1930s and 1940s were transferred to radiation protection and civil defence in the 1950s.[22] As early as 1950, the Ministry of the Interior convened an advisory committee for civil defence in the event of a nuclear war. Physicists and radiologists discussed ways of protecting the population and the emergency services from the threat of radioactivity. In 1955, the government established the "Deutsche Atomkommission" (German Atomic Commission) – the main advisory body for nuclear research and industries. In 1957, the "Sonderausschuß Radioaktivität," responsible for radiation monitoring in West Germany, started work. The commissions established sub-committees for radiation-measuring instruments. The state became actively involved in instrument manufacturing. The committees co-ordinated technological developments, distributed information on the trade and determined instrument specifications required for civil defence.[23] The scientists represented in the commissions managed the crucial link between instrument design and specific concepts of radiation protection.

Germany imported mainly American-made radiation-measuring instruments until domestic manufacturers managed to construct practical instruments. In the early 1950s, a large number of companies entered the field of nuclear instrumentation. They were drawn from the electrotechnical industry, for example Siemens (Karlsruhe); the radiographic industry, for example "Laboratorium Prof. Dr. Berthold" (Wildbad); or the radio industry, for example "Frieseke & Hoepfner" (Erlangen), to name but a few influential companies. In 1959, a government directory listed 53 manufacturers of nuclear instruments in Germany.[24] Separation of the development of instruments from the practice of experimental physics effectively evolved in Germany in the early 1950s. The companies became an independent factor in nuclear politics. At the same time, it was necessary to co-ordinate industrial production, nuclear research and government regulations. A government advisory committee dealt exclusively with the design of radiation-measuring instruments. The committee's chairman, Wolfgang Gentner, from 1949 Professor of Physics in Freiburg and later in Heidelberg, established a large collection of foreign instruments that influenced the specifications for the design of instruments in West Germany.[25] In addition, the nuclear research centres equipped electronic laboratories for the development of instruments and the standardisation of nuclear instrumentation. However, in contrast to some American research centres, they did not produce large series of equipment, but restricted their efforts to industrial advice.[26] The manufacturers themselves established close links with the nuclear research centres; their presence became most obvious in courses on the practice of radiation measurement that provided opportunities for future users to become accustomed to the instruments.

In the 1950s, the atomic nucleus caught the attention of many different groups: physicists, politicians in the Federal Government and the federal states, instrument manufacturers, employees in nuclear industries, the military, the emergency services and the so-called lay public. The atom appeared to be the universal answer to all problems of public and private life. It brought the promise of health and wealth as well as a solution for the problems of transportation and energy.[27] At the same time, nuclear hazards fundamentally changed both working conditions and private life. Regulations concerning radiation protection were set in place in order to maintain an awareness of safety. It is not my task here to evaluate the effectiveness of different approaches to radiation protection; instead, I will outline general arguments that appeared as plausible means of establishing a definition of safety in the presence of radiation hazards. The various approaches to the realisation of safety differed in the specific responsibilities they attributed to scientific experts, state authorities, protection crews, sections of the population affected, and measuring instruments.

Radiation in the Workplace

In post-war Germany, radiation endangered an increasing number of employees. Since the first deliveries of isotopes in 1948, the handling of radioactive substances had become part of the day-to-day experiences of scientists and employees in medicine, industry and agriculture. According to numbers produced by the unions, more than 70,000 workers were exposed to radioactivity in 1957.[28] Before the Second World War, the risk of exposure had been regulated within the professions concerned; after the Second World War, a changing public perception of radiation and the increase in the number of people handling radioactivity led to state regulation. In addition, the US authorities insisted on the imposition of legal regulations before Germany could count on the delivery of American nuclear fuels.[29] Public promotion of the nuclear industries was paralleled by legislation and support for instrument-manufacturing industry. From 1956, the scientists and civil servants of the German Atomic Commission discussed regulations on radiation protection; in 1957, the Federal Government began to prepare a decree on radiation protection that was finally promulgated in 1960. It is important to emphasise that, while politicians generally acknowledged the need for tough regulations, this did not imply that they had fundamental doubts about the benefits of nuclear energy – they saw the regulations as means of promoting the new technology. They argued that the lack of regulations at the beginning of the Industrial Revolution had led to pollution; they therefore insisted on investing in safety measures right at the beginning of the Nuclear Age. It is not sufficient to dismiss these considerations as mere "safety rhetoric." Although the radiation protection decree remained controversial, it provided guidelines for "safe" working conditions that could be adhered to. In public, physicists frequently claimed that workplace safety in the nuclear industries was superior to that in the chemical industry, for example. They justified their claims by referring to tighter regulations and more sensitive radiation detectors.[30] Thus, instruments concerned with radiation formed an indispensible contribution to the image of safe nuclear industries.

Regulations at a local level supplemented, and sometimes even pre-dated, state legislation that was implemented in 1960. In the late 1950s, nuclear research centres established special measurement departments to enforce safety regulations. They enjoyed particular independence from management and were authorised to intervene in experiments if radiation safety was endangered. Objects for radiation protection also filled isotope laboratories. Shields and containers protected radioactive materials, and special tools made it possible for researchers to work at a distance from the source of radiation. Such measures had already been the cornerstone of regulations before the Second World War.[31] In addition, measuring instruments

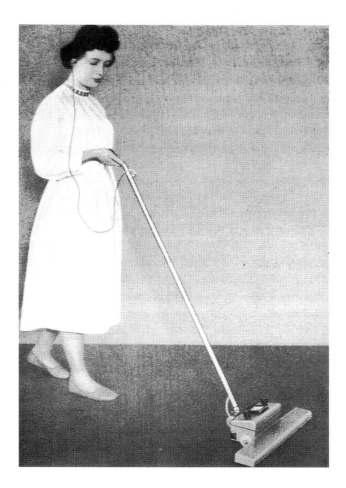

Figure 2. Advertisement for a contamination monitor [Mitteilungsblätter Strahlungsmeßgeräte (Frieseke & Hoepfner, Erlangen), *1 (1960): 10].*

surrounded employees in radiation laboratories. Measurements in the workplace became regular practice. Film badges and dosimeters registered the doses of radiation to which workers were exposed, and portable contamination monitors enabled the detection of local contamination. In order to measure confined radioactive sources without exposing the employees to full radiation, Geiger–Müller tubes were fixed to poles. These devices combined two principles of radiation protection: taking measurements, and keeping a distance from the potential source of radiation. The separation of detector and control panel is a manifestation of the basic principle of radiation protection: keep your distance![32]

Regulations instructed the employees how to behave in the hazardous environment: eating, drinking and smoking were forbidden. The workplace had to be clean and tidy. In case of contamination, it was the duty of employees to clean the areas thoroughly. The progress of decontamination had to be checked with radiation-measuring instruments.[33]

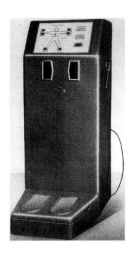

Figure 3. Advertisement for a hand and foot monitor [Mitteilungsblätter Strahlungsmeßgeräte (Frieseke & Hoepfner, Erlangen), *3 (1960): 14].*

Instructions demanding care and order were an integral part of all regulations concerned with radiation protection. "Hoover"-shaped Geiger counters might have been a reminder of the cleanliness required (*see* Figure 2). Care and order not only reduced health hazards, but also prevented the malfunction of instruments as a result of contamination. Instructions on cleanliness and discipline at work put the onus of responsibility on the workers. Authorities in the nuclear industry identified carelessness, thoughtlessness and negligence as the prime causes of injuries.[34] Measuring instruments not only detected radiation, but also ensured care and order – the instruments became indicators of the character of the workers.

Concepts of radiation protection relied not only on the employees' personal responsibility, but also on work organisation and workplace layout. Protection regulations defined areas in which exposure to radiation might exceed a certain limit as "control areas." Early proposals for the West German radiation protection act used the term "danger zone;" atomic ministry experts rejected this and introduced the terms "control area" and "warning area."[35] This terminology was chosen in order to calm the worries of the employees, but it does also reflect the conviction that technological control made it possible to avoid dangers. "Danger" was not perceived as an inherent quality of these workplaces, but rather as a unique event in the case of accidents. Technical control reduced the possibility of accidents; technical warning allowed the workers to escape danger.

Before leaving control areas, employees were obliged to check for contamination. The location of personnel monitors became a characteristic of zones with high radiation risks. The instruments dictated the structure of the nuclear workplace. The layout of research centres afforded a clear distinction between safe and hazardous areas.[36] Radiation monitors detected the contamination of workers' hands, shoes and bodies (*see* Figure 3). Alarms indicated excessive counts. Further alarms ensured that the person whose contamination was being measured remained for the prescribed time of measurement.[37] A "Doorpost Gamma Radiation Monitor" was able to detect the movement of a reasonably strong radioactive source through a doorway; it comprised two Geiger–Müller counters on either side of the doorway. These counters registered any dramatic increase over the background level of radiation and could thus identify a contaminated worker as a radiation source and sound the alarm.

Regulations concerned with radiation protection rested on the concept of a "tolerance dose." Biophysicists and politicians at the highest level agreed that the tolerance dose was no more than a disguise for the practice of changing scientific conventions without sufficient experimental evidence. The Minister of Atomic Energy, Siegfried Balke, even called the tolerance dose a threshold to calm the public and workers concerned.[38] The tolerance dose defined a reference threshold for safe working conditions; it was a practical way of establishing "safety" that went beyond individual evaluation and experience. Radiation-measuring instruments sustained occupational safety – they proved that radiation was within the officially defined limit. The alarms on these devices can be seen as a manifestation of this method of dealing with health hazards by defining thresholds.[39]

Workplace safety was closely related to the organisation of the research centres. As a result of this, prevention of accidents was the responsibility of the leadership. The Minister of Atomic Energy emphasised in 1957 that every injury proved mismanagement and a lack of leadership. Radiation-measuring instruments not only controlled discipline at work, but also placed responsibility for the safety of the employees with the management.[40]

The instruments described so far were part of the system of radiation protection in large nuclear research centres and reactors. In general, industrial users of isotopes did not have these instruments at their disposal, therefore the federal states of West Germany established radiation-measuring crews. The factory inspectorate or the employment ministry equipped radiation-measuring cars that travelled around, making the prescribed measurements.[41]

Concepts of workshop safety relied on regulations that provided standards for "safe" working conditions. Authorised crews supervised work that involved radioactive substances. The enforcement of safety regulations depended on measuring instruments that structured both the work organisation of the management *and* the work practice of the individual employees.

Fallout and Radiation Safety

Nuclear research centres appeared to be sources of danger, not only to their employees, but also for people living near reactors. Safety, therefore, was not only an issue within the nuclear workplace, but had also to be established outside in the local environment. Physicists managing reactor projects calmed the concerns of the state governments by explaining the automatic radiation surveillance of reactors. They argued that radiation leaks were extremely improbable, but, even if a leak occurred, the Geiger counter would indicate it immediately. Health physics departments surveyed the areas surrounding nuclear research centres; stationary instruments monitored radiation in water, in the atmosphere and in soil. These radiation measurements allowed for the monitoring of the as-yet-unknown behaviour of reactors.[42]

The health physics department of the Nuclear Research Centre in Karlsruhe had a van at their disposal. It was equipped with a large measuring instrument, a recorder, a scintillation counter, a small portable counter, and chemical devices for the preparation of plants and water before measurements. The radiation monitors for such investigations consisted of several modules (*see* Figure 4). The manufacturing industry offered a range of counting tubes, pulse amplifiers and registration devices. Such a modular construction system made possible the adaptation of measuring instruments to meet the specific needs of the laboratories.[43]

It was the task of these instruments to prove the *absence* of radiation released by nuclear reactors. At the same time, these radiation measurements demonstrated the *presence* of radiation in the atmosphere resulting from nuclear fallout after atomic bomb testing. In 1953, Otto Haxel (Heidelberg University) and Wolfgang Gentner (Freiburg University) and their colleagues had already begun measuring radioactivity in the atmosphere and in rain. These measurements were an important source of information about nuclear-weapons testing for the West German Government. The physics department of Freiburg University became the Central Office for radioactive fallout; it published regular reports, starting in 1956. The measurements revealed a drastic increase in radiation, which was publicly perceived as a danger to the health of the population. The measurements, which were originally intended as a source of information on the risks involved in a nuclear war, became evidence of a possible threat even in peacetime.[44]

The German Government ordered the permanent registration of radiation. Between 1955 and 1960, an expanding network of instruments made the national surveillance of radiation possible. A number of state institutions at regional and national levels, several university departments and private institutes monitored radiation in the atmosphere, in water and in food. This multitude of measurements was an ideal basis for disagreement. Controversies about radiation measurements were a frequent source of conflict between scientists of various disciplines and state authorities. The headline of a Munich tabloid read: "Controversy on Contaminated Water Brought New Surprise: Even Our Milk is in Danger. Two Authorities in Dispute."[45] Several strategies were available to deal with and reduce these uncertainties: the unification of methods, the centralisation of measurements and the development of standardised measuring techniques. Scientists called for state intervention to standardise the methods.[46] In addition, government officials proposed to authorise only those state institutions equipped to undertake the surveillance of radiation, while university departments were to be concerned with developing new measuring technologies. The argument was that radiation monitoring was a task of the state and therefore should be controlled by the state; the authorisation of state institutions to measure radiation was an attempt to provide uncontroversial data. The Federal Government consequently supported a network of measuring stations all over the country. Water supply companies and meteorological services were the first to measure radiation in the atmosphere and in waste water both systematically and continuously. In 1955, the German Weather Service was given responsibility for monitoring the atmosphere, to supplement the activities of the institutions that were already in charge of radiation measurements in water, food and in the soil. The permanent registration of radiation was seen as a means to avert hazards to human life.

These institutes were occupied with routine measurements that had previously been the task of physicists who, from the beginnings of their careers, had been accustomed to making measurements of radiation, and who consequently frequently emphasised their skills in evaluating the quality of measurements. The expansion of responsibility for routine measurements increased the number of less-qualified people being involved in the determination of radiation. Meteorologists, biologists and other scientists employed in institutions instructed to monitor radiation struggled with the unfamiliar task. As a result, new requirements emerged for the measuring technologies. In order to overcome the restrictions presented by the working hours of assistants reading the instruments, the devices were equipped with automatic recorders. The construction of devices with long-term reliability became a new challenge for the instrument manufacturing industry; scientists frequently complained about instruments that worked properly for only a couple of weeks. At first, the German Weather Service was equipped with automatically registering instruments from Switzerland. They used Swiss instruments because German counters counted unreliably and thereby required supervision by trained people; the Swiss instruments, in contrast, were "foolproof."[47] While academic scientists relied on their individual expertise when they judged the proper working of measuring devices, reliably working instruments were seen as a guarantee of competent measurements performed by non-specialists.

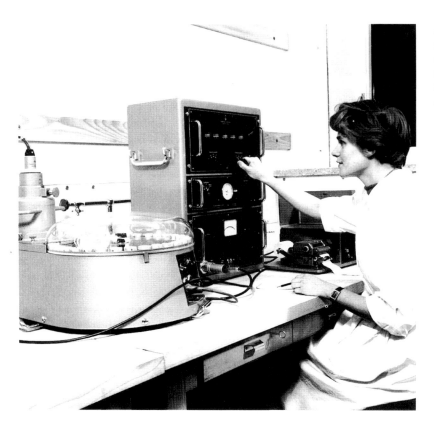

Figure 4. Large radiation monitor FH 49 of Frieseke & Hoepfner (Erlangen) in the radiation biology department of the Nuclear Research Centre Karlsruhe, 1958.

The need for qualified judgement when assessing the potential hazard of radiation was an obstacle for non-experts. Instruments automatically indicated an increase in radiation beyond a certain threshold. However, the determination of total radiation was not sufficient for the assessment of health hazards. Radiologists took into account radiation only from those elements with half-lives sufficiently long to be of significance; measuring devices automated the complex laboratory processes involved in these evaluations. Standardised measuring technologies reduced the need for expert judgement that tended to be a source of disagreement.[48]

In the 1950s, the government had thus reacted to the awareness of radiation hazards in the atmosphere and on the ground, in water and in food, with the establishment of a network of measuring offices. This extension of routine measurements brought about changes in the design of measuring instruments. Long-term reliability, further automation and standardisation of data evaluation became requirements for measuring devices. The network of measuring offices and instruments monitoring radiation in the environment afforded proof of the provision of care by the government and thereby established "safety" in everyday life.

The Geiger Counter and Civil Defence

While radiation in the workplace and nuclear fallout became part of everyday life, radioactive contamination caused by a nuclear war preoccupied the imaginations of politicians and rescue teams. The possible exposure of a large number of people to high levels of radiation required strategies for the protection of the entire population. As a result of this extension of the scope of protection measures, it became necessary to involve non-scientists in radiation measurements. For this reason, the question of expertise gained particular significance. The nature of the instruments reflected this problem, and was closely related to civil defence organisation. In 1953, the Ministry of the Interior considered supplying the entire population with small dosimeters that registered individual doses of radiation. These instruments – film badges or ball-pen ionisation chambers – allowed control of atomic hazards with reference to individual radiation exposure. The scientists on the committee for radiation instruments considered in detail the problem of whether the instruments should have an open display. Every user would have had access to immediate information on his or her exposure to radiation; open access to the data was seen as a potential source of panic. For that reason, the consultant scientists favoured devices *documenting* the dose; *evaluation* of the measurements should be a responsibility restricted to centralised radiation offices.[49] In this way, it was possible to limit access to the information that could be deduced from the instruments.

For practical and financial reasons, the committee decided to equip only emergency services personnel with individual dosimeters, and not the entire population. Instead of requiring *individual* exposure to be monitored,

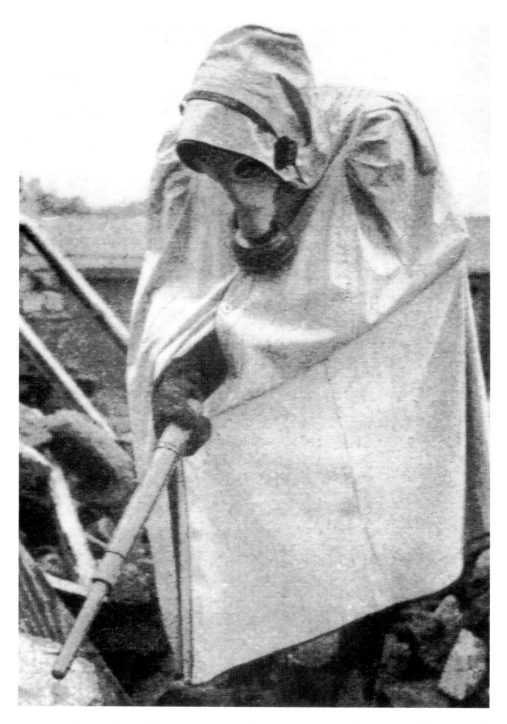

Figure 5. Air-raid drill with radiation measuring instrument in 1959 [Bundesluftschutzverband Köln (ed.), Lehrbuch für leitende Helfer und Luftschutzlehrer im Bundesluftschutzverband. *Vol. 1.* Selbsthilfe im Zivilen Luftschutz. *(Cologne, 1959), p. 27].*

the committee approved the surveillance of *areas* affected by a nuclear attack. The Geiger–Müller counter was particularly suitable for this task; the choice of the instrument was based on a specific concept of radiation protection in civil defence: the control of contaminated areas (in contrast to the alternative concept of monitoring the individual dose). The instruments became a characteristic of those specialised teams in charge of maintaining the health and safety of the population should a nuclear war occur. It was the job of measuring crews to mark radioactive areas and determine the permissible duration of stay. These applications required tough, portable instruments that were water resistant and, above all, easy to operate. Figure 5 shows a portable instrument for the detection of radiation: the counting tube and the amplifier were fitted in a bar, and the pulses were registered acoustically using earphones. One did not need much training to take the measurements; however, in order to assess the hazards, one had to gain some practical experience in interpreting the clicks in the earphone: it was a matter of personal evaluation and judgement to infer radiation threats from the acoustic signals.[50]

Such rough-and-ready measurements of radiation based on the personal experience of the measuring crews were generally unsatisfactory. Strategies of civil defence relied on quantitative values that prescribed further action. The duration of permissible stay in a contaminated area, for example, depended on calculations that took into consideration the tolerance dose and the activity in the region. Quantitative measurements required specially qualified crews. The scientists on the committee on radiation protection still believed the scientific terms such as "dose" or "dose rate" to be too complex for members of the emergency services. For this reason, they considered producing instruments that immediately indicated the time of permissible stay: in ambiguous situations – when the protection crews were confronted with the conflicting values of self-protection versus the protection of others and of inanimate objects – the instruments allowed fast decisions as to restriction of access to contaminated areas.

Members of emergency services were expected to make decisions on rescue attempts affecting health and survival of citizens in the face of nuclear contamination. The commission on civil defence aimed at a reduction of individual evaluation and judgement. They defined the amount of radiation to which members of protection crews were permitted to be exposed. They allowed, not only for the possibility of health defects, but also for the problem of decreasing human efficiency as a result of exposure to radiation. They struggled with the dilemma that every rescue attempt in a contaminated area presented a radiation hazard for the protection crew. State institutions settled these problems by creating rules and making decrees.[51] The design of instruments for civil defence was adapted to these regulations, in order to provide a clear basis for further action. Their range of sensitivity and the design of the instrumental scales depended on previously determined threshold values. Concealing the complex negotiations surrounding the matter of the so-called tolerance dose, the instruments provided clear-cut data in accordance with prescribed regulations.

In addition to portable radiation-measuring instruments, central radiation laboratories were equipped with instruments for the measurement of radiation in water, air, dust and food. In contrast to the instruments mentioned above, the use of these devices and the complex evaluation of the data they generated required special training.[52] The Ministry of the Interior suggested equipping a mobile measuring station with large radiation-measuring instruments; the civil servants favoured mobile stations because stationary instruments could be endangered in the event of a nuclear attack. In addition, the German Red Cross kept two measuring vans for use in disasters caused by accidents in nuclear reactors. These various measuring vans allowed the surveillance of radiation to be made independently of stationary laboratories.[53]

The press frequently published reports about super-bombs and impending nuclear war. These articles portrayed the population as defencelessly exposed to the invisible and deadly dust that could be detected only with a Geiger counter.[54] In such situations, the public was told, they should trust radiation crews tracing radioactive contamination with Geiger counters. Measuring radiation was presented as a means of controlling it. Although the emergency services used a variety of different instruments, in public, the Geiger counter became the the device that characterised rescue teams controlling radiation.

Safety in case of a nuclear war relied on specialised crews mastering measuring instruments. These objects brought about a hierarchical structure within the civil defence services that was linked to the application of different classes of radiation-measuring instruments: the lay public did not have any instruments; members of protection crews were equipped with small dosimeters, several radiation detectors and dose-rate meters; and finally, specialised officers managed the most sensitive and advanced instruments. This hierarchy in civil defence also emerged from the means of decision making. The kind of information available to the various groups depended both on the instruments and on the conclusions that could be drawn from the measurements. Some devices suggested formal, strictly rule-governed decisions with hardly any scope for judgement, while others provided data amenable only to expert evaluation and judgement.

The Volks-Geiger Counter

The expanding network of measuring instruments proved the ubiquity of radiation. In addition, in the early years of the Cold War, nuclear war was a permanent threat. The different sources of nuclear hazards blurred in the perception of politicians and the press. This had enormous consequences for the meanings that were ascribed to radiation-measuring instruments.

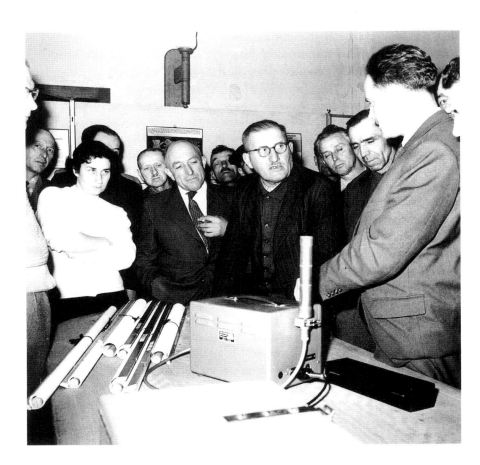

Figure 6. Public Information meeting organised by the Nuclear Research Centre Karlsruhe, 1957.

It is interesting to examine the effect of the Geiger counter on the relationship between the public, scientists and civil servants. First, it is necessary to spend some time considering how politicians perceived the public's reaction to radiation in their day-to-day life. Since the early 1950s, the German tabloids regularly reported on fallout and the contamination of the environment and of food. In the view of most politicians and scientists, these reports distorted the proper purpose of scientific articles on this issue and caused unnecessary public concern. Civil servants of the Atomic Ministry frequently labelled the reactions of the public as a "radiation psychosis."[55] A government adviser identified the public's difficulty in *perceiving* radiation as being the origin of the "magic," "irrational," "emotional" fears of the population. He demanded that the public had to be convinced that radiation was not an unknown, unpredictable, magic power, but a natural force that could be controlled by scientific experts.[56] It is important to emphasise that it was in the government's interest to inform the population regularly concerning radiation. The government saw the need to "accustom the German population to radiation hazards." This information had to be accompanied by confirmation that the government had taken measures for the public's protection.[57]

The health physics department of the Nuclear Research Centre in Karlsruhe complained about the increasing public doubts caused by the black-and-white portrayal of press reports on nuclear-weapons tests.[58] Confronted with opposition from villages in the neighbourhood of the planned reactor near Karlsruhe, the Nuclear Research Centre organised meetings at which the public was informed about how the reactor worked. The Geiger counter shown in Figure 6 was one of the few original instruments they brought with them. This instrument represented the entire network of measuring installations that spanned the research centre and the surrounding area. Furthermore, the radiation-measuring department demanded that measurements should be undertaken publicly, so that the people were able to convince themselves of the safety of the reactor. The van with the instruments driving through the villages around the reactor not only measured the radioactivity in the entire neighbourhood, but also demonstrated, by the visible presence of the counting tube on the roof, the ubiquity of the safety network and its operation (*see* Figure 7). It was the achievement of the Geiger counter that it registered a potential danger – and thereby created safety.[59]

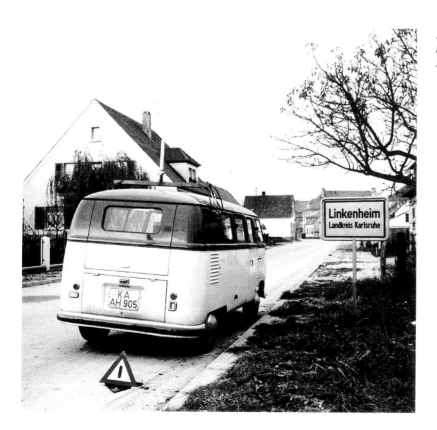

Figure 7. Measuring minibus of the Nuclear Research Centre Karlsruhe, 1957.

Why shouldn't everybody be able to own a Geiger counter? Since the late 1950s, many manufacturers of radiation-measuring instruments considered the production of a so-called "Volksgeigerzähler" – a people's counter. The discourse about instruments controlling radiation was embodied in the new artefact of the Volks-Geiger counter. The instrument fitted into strategies for personal radiation protection that had already been discussed in relation to the field of civil defence. In contrast to the personal dosimeters mentioned above, the Volks-Geiger counter relied on the idea of a responsible citizen mastering information regarding the contamination of the environment and of food. At the beginning of the 1960s, many manufacturers of measuring instruments anticipated a growing market for these instruments. Some even considered marketing small radiation monitors via the popular mail-order firm, Neckermann.

Emergency services had already been equipped with small, portable Geiger–Müller counters. At the beginning of the 1960s, the federal states supplied several offices with small, portable instruments.[60] However, the production of Volks-Geiger counters went far beyond the concepts embodied in these instruments for disaster control: they satisfied both the demand of government officials organising civil defence and the desire of the public to gain access to information about radiation in their day-to-day life. The government supported this idea of broadening the range of users of radiation-measuring instruments.

Similar devices were produced by a manufacturer of cameras, AGFA; the instrument could be kept in a camera box, and the earphones were stored in a camera-case lens-pocket.[61] A prime requirement for such counters was that they should be affordable: they were priced in the range DM100–150. The Ministry of the Interior welcomed their development. Of particular interest were counters installed in transistor radios – government officials hoped such a combination would increase the popularity of the measuring instruments.[62]

The Volks-Geiger counter was seen as an instrument that would give the lay public the ability to control radiation hazards in food and in the environment – a task that had previously been restricted to scientists. The press reported eagerly on new developments: the headline of a paper in Augsburg read: "First Lively Dance Music – Then the Geiger Counter Clicks. Pocket-sized Radio is Radiation Measuring Instrument."[63] The national press also praised the invention of Volks-Geiger counters. The *Frankfurter Allgemeine Zeitung* reported: "Radiation Measurements Made Easy."[64] The article claimed that the counter could be used like a radio, without any expert knowledge.

Scientific experts firmly rejected the concept of the Volks-Geiger counter, insisting on the complex laboratory equipment needed to assess the health hazards of radioactive contamination. They judged the simple testing of food to be insufficient for the evaluation of potential threats. Health physicists at the Nuclear Research Centre in Karlsruhe emphasised: "The individual is unable to judge the real hazard of contamination. Even the

Volks-Geiger counter can't change that."[65] The scientists in charge of radiation protection were well aware of the constraints of their job; they knew of the complexity and ambiguity of radiation measurements; they understood that the assessment of health hazards and the definition of radiation safety depended on conventions maintained by institutions that regulated decision-making processes. Scientists thus defended their role as experts in radiation matters, referring to the *social nature* of their judgements – social in the sense that the evaluation of hazards depended on institutional agreements, which were without complete scientific evidence and open to permanent revision. In contrast, the press and government officials promoting the use of Volks-Geiger counters perceived the problem of safety as clear-cut, considering that it could be settled using a simple instrument. From this point of view, radiation safety was reduced to the *technological problem* of registering radiation: individuals were in charge of controlling, and thereby maintaining, safety.

It might be worth emphasising that there were no regulations as to how to act in case of increased radiation. Scientists of the German Atomic Commission were unhappy that the population had no information about protection measures. Riezler, the chairman of the Protection Commission, and Otto Haxel, scientist at Heidelberg University, supported this point with very drastic arguments referring to the nuclear incident in 1954, when some fishermen on Bikini Atoll were caught in nuclear fallout. That entire affair had received extensive press coverage in Germany, as it was the first time that the global effects of radiation and its global threat became public. Haxel argued that the serious illness of the Bikini fishermen was caused by their ignorance of any protection measures – they had eaten contaminated fish. He claimed that similar incidents could happen in Germany if the population was not informed of protection measures that they could take.[66] The Volks-Geiger counter did not solve this problem; it served only to prove the presence of radiation in food and in the environment.

The instruments were not a success on the market. The Ministry of the Interior gave up its proposals to distribute them for the purpose of civil defence because of the high costs involved; the manufacturers complained about slow sales; atomic scientists questioned the use of the instruments on principle. However, their production is testimony to the belief in the power of instruments to provide a safety control for everybody.

Conclusion

In order to assess the significance of the Geiger counter in the twentieth century, it is essential to understand its use for public regulation and control. A range of institutions involving government officials, scientists, instrument manufacturers and the emergency services "settled" the problem of radiation safety – they provided practical guidelines and arguments that allowed them to speak of safety in the presence of radiation hazards. Nuclear war, radiation in the workplace and radioactive fallout required different safety measures. In each case, measuring instruments reflected the debates on specific features of radiation protection. It was a question of *social order* to designate those who were in charge of radiation control. The design of the instruments became a crucial factor in the organisation of protection measures. The qualifications necessary for making measurements, and the information obtainable, depended on the instruments. Instruments such as large radiation monitors (Figure 5) embodied the concept of qualified-expert systems with exclusive access to data. In contrast, the Volks-Geiger counter represented the ideal of responsible citizens with free access to information.

Radiation-measuring instruments made the application of safety regulations possible. The devices were adapted for day-to-day measurements and thus dictated *control procedures*. The determination of threshold values marking the boundary between safety and danger was of crucial significance for radiation control. Contemporary physicists and radiologists emphasised that the definitions of "threshold values," of "admissible exposure to radiation" and of "radiation safety" relied on changing scientific conventions. In common with atomic radiation itself, these conventions could not be experienced in day-to-day life. However, the definition of threshold values transformed the problem of safety into the technical problem of determining the level of radiation.

The Geiger–Müller counter was not only an important instrument for radiation control. By reference to the Geiger counter, it was possible to represent the entire network of instruments and institutions controlling radiation. However, the *symbolic meaning* of the instruments went beyond a visible exemplification of authorities enforcing safety standards. In 1956, a newspaper emphasised that no-one denied the danger of radioactivity. However, "as soon as it is possible to grasp a danger, its dangerous face disappears."[67] The Geiger counter's impressive representation of radiation publicly demonstrated the capacity to control radioactivity. In the 1950s, it was a widely held belief that the *detection* of radiation was a means to create *safety*. By the late 1960s, this attitude had changed – and measurements came to be representative of danger, rather than to be perceived as creating safety.

Notes

This work was funded by grants from the Volkswagen Stiftung and the Deutscher Akademischer Austauschdienst. Many thanks to those who have been a source of ideas, criticism and practical help: Martina Blum, Alexander Gall, Jeff Hughes, Jürgen Lieske, Gerhard Mener, Barbara Schmucki, Helmuth Trischler, Ulrich Wengenroth, Thomas Wieland, Thomas Zeller, Clemens Zimmermann. The audience and commentators of earlier presentations of the paper provided useful criticisms. Not being a native English speaker, I relied on the help of Eve Duffy, Alex and David Williams for the revision of the paper. I would like to thank the following institutions for providing illustrations: Forschungszentrum Karlsruhe, Stabsabteilung Öffentlichkeitsarbeit, Postfach 3640, D-76021 Karlsruhe; Deutsches Museum München, Bildstelle, D-80306 München.

1. "Sind wir schon radioaktiv verseucht? Geigerzähler auf der Alm," *Hamburger Abendblatt*, September 21, 1956.
2. "In einem Glas Wein oder einer Tasse Milch steckt nicht der Tod," *Hamburger Abendblatt*, September 21, 1956.
3. Hans A. Künkel, *Atomschutzfibel. Die deutsche Wissenschaft urteilt* (Göttingen, 1950), p. 37; "Geigerzähler auf der Alm" (n. 1 above).
4. D. Alan Bromley, "Evolution and Use of Nuclear Detectors and Systems," *Nuclear Instruments and Methods* 162 (1979): 1.
5. My considerations on the social effects of artefacts follow closely a more general argument in Michael Shanks and Christopher Tilley, *Re-Constructing Archaeology. Theory and Practice* (Cambridge, 1987), pp. 133–34. See also Steven Lubar and David Kingery, eds, *History from Things. Essays on Material Culture* (Washington, 1993).
6. Gabrielle Hecht has recently provided an analysis of artefacts in the nuclear workplace regarding the practice of risk management in relation to broader social, cultural and political issues. See Gabrielle Hecht, "Rebels and Pioneers. Technocratic Ideologies and Social Identities in the French Nuclear Workplace, 1955–1969," *Social Studies of Science* 26 (1996): 483–530.
7. The early history of the invention of the Geiger–Müller counter is well known, see Thaddeus J. Trenn, "The Geiger–Müller Counter of 1928," *Annals of Science* 43 (1986): 111–36, and Friedrich G. Rheingans, *Hans Geiger und die elektrischen Zählmethoden, 1908–1928* (Berlin, 1988).
8. See for example Hans Geiger and Walther Müller, "Das Elektronenzählrohr," *Physikalische Zeitschrift* 29 (1928): 839–41; letter of Walther Müller to his parents, July 26, 1928, Deutsches Museum, Archiv, NL 24–7/30.
9. Rheingans (n. 7 above), p. 42; see also the correspondence between Müller and his parents 1928–1929, the letter about Bohr's visit to Kiel is dated June 20, 1929, Deutsches Museum, Archiv, NL 24–7/30. On Geiger's popularity as a public lecturer, see Edgar Swinne, *Hans Geiger. Spuren aus einem Leben für die Physik* (Berlin, 1988), pp. 84–85.
10. Jeff Hughes, "The Radioactivists. Community, Controversy and the Rise of Nuclear Physics" (Ph.D. diss., Cambridge University, 1993); Jeff Hughes, "Plasticine and Valves. Industry, Instrumentation and the Emergence of Nuclear Physics," in *The Invisible Industrialist. Manufactures and the Construction of Scientific Knowledge*, ed. J. P. Gaudillère, I. Lowy, and D. Pestre (London, 1997). On the automation of measurements, see also Hans Geiger, "Der Einfluß der Atomphysik auf unser Weltbild," in *Deutschland in der Wende der Zeiten [Öffentliche Vorträge der Universität Tübingen, Sommersemester 1933]* (Stuttgart, 1934), p. 113, and Walther Bothe, "Die Geigerschen Zählmethoden," *Die Naturwissenschaften* 30 (1942): 596.
11. Hughes, "The Radioactivists" (n. 10 above), has provided an excellent analysis of the emergence of a nuclear physics community in relation to changing experimental instruments and practices. See also Jeff Hughes, "The French Connection. 'Nuclear Physics' in Paris 1928–1932," *History and Technology*, Special Issue (forthcoming); Peter Galison, *How Experiments End* (Chicago, 1987), pp. 75–133. On the history of the German atomic bomb project, see Mark Walker, *German National Socialism and the Quest for Nuclear Power, 1939–1949* (Cambridge, 1989) and Richard Rhodes, *The Making of the Atomic Bomb* (London, 1988).
12. "Universitätsinstitut für physikalische Grundlagen der Medizin."
13. Boris Rajewsky, "Physikalische Diagnostik der Radiumvergiftungen. Einrichtung einer Untersuchungsstelle," *Strahlentherapie* 69 (1941): 438–502. On radium poisoning in the USA, see Catharine Caufield, *Multiple Exposures. Chronicles of the Radiation Age* (London, 1989), pp. 29–40.
14. On the changes in medical practice related to the introduction of the stethoscope, see Jens Lachmund, "Die Erfindung des ärztlichen Gehörs. Zur historischen Soziologie der stethoskopischen Untersuchung," *Zeitschrift für Soziologie* 21 (1992): 235–51.
15. Rajewsky (n. 13 above). See also Boris Rajewsky, "On the Development of Devices for the Determination of Total-Body Radioactivity in Man," in *Assessment of Radioactivity in Man. Proceedings of the Symposium held by the International Atomic Energy Agency at Heidelberg (May 11–16, 1964)*, vol. 1 (Vienna, 1964), pp. 15–52.
16. Boris Rajewsky, "Das Geiger–Müller-Zählrohr im Dienste des Bergbaus," *Zeitschrift für Physik* 120 (1943): 627–38.

17. Erwin Fünfer, "Zählrohrsuchgerät zur Auffindung verlorenen Radiums," *Die Umschau* 43 (1939): 304.

18. On Operation Paperclip see, for example, Tom Bower, *The Paperclip Conspiracy. The Battle for the Spoils and Secrets of Nazi Germany* (London, 1987) and Anne-Lydia Edingshaus, *Heinz Maier-Leibnitz – ein halbes Jahrhundert experimentelle Physik* (München, 1986).

19. On the lack of scientific co-operation in Germany, see *Operation Epsilon. The Farm Hall Transcripts. Introduced by Sir Charles Frank* (Bristol/Philadelphia, 1993), p. 70 ff. On the idea of "falling behind" see Bernd A. Rusinek, *Das Forschungszentrum. Eine Geschichte der KFA Jülich von ihrer Gründung bis 1980* [*Studien zur Geschichte der deutschen Großforschungseinrichtungen* Bd. 11] (Frankfurt/New York, 1996), pp. 203–15.

20. A sample of the extensive literature on West German nuclear industries: Joachim Radkau, *Aufstieg und Krise der deutschen Atomwirtschaft. 1945–1975. Verdrängte Alternativen in der Kerntechnik und der Ursprung der nuklearen Kontroverse* (Reinbek, 1983); Wolfgang D. Müller, *Geschichte der Kernenergie in der Bundesrepublik Deutschland. Anfänge und Weichenstellungen* (Stuttgart, 1990); Michael Eckert and Maria Osietzki, *Wissenschaft für Markt und Macht. Kernforschung und Mikroelektronik in der Bundesrepublik Deutschland* (München, 1989). Several detailed studies of nuclear research centres resulted from a project on the history of large scale research in West Germany; for further references, see Margit Szöllösi-Janze and Helmuth Trischler, eds., *Großforschung in Deutschland* [*Studien zur Geschichte der deutschen Großforschungseinrichtungen* Bd. 1] (Frankfurt, 1990); Rusinek (n. 19 above).

21. Spencer R. Weart, *Scientists in Power* (Cambridge, Mass., 1979).

22. Pre-war nuclear physicists and biophysicists became leading figures in the committees for nuclear instrumentation and radiation protection: Wolfgang Riezler, Boris Rajewsky, Walther Bothe, Walther Gerlach. Students and research assistants of Hans Geiger and his close colleague Walther Bothe were well represented: Wolfgang Gentner, Heinz Maier-Leibnitz, Otto Haxel, Christian Gerthsen, to name only a few influential members of the committees.

23. On the history of the "Deutsche Atomkommission" see Radkau (n. 20 above), pp. 137–48.

24. "Alphabetisches Firmen- und Warengruppenverzeichnis," January 1, 1959, Bundesarchiv Koblenz B 138/256.

25. Bundesarchiv Koblenz B 106/17176–17178.

26. See for example "Prof. Friedburg: Konzept für die Zukunft des Labors für Elektronik," Generallandesarchiv Karlsruhe 69–1024.

27. The promises of peaceful uses of atomic energy emerged from the older belief in the power of large technical projects to provide universal solutions, see Alexander Gall, *Das Atlantropaprojekt* (Frankfurt, 1998). See also Bernd-A. Rusinek, "'Kernenergie, schöner Götterfunken!' Die 'umgekehrte Demontage'. Zur Kontextgeschichte der Atomeuphorie," *Kultur & Technik* 17, no. 4 (1993): 15–21; Rusinek (n. 19 above), pp. 89–120.

28. Correspondence Deutscher Gewerkschaftsbund–Atomministerium, May 15, 1957, Bundesarchiv Koblenz B 138/570.

29. On radiation protection before the Second World War, see Daniel Paul Serwer, "The Rise of Radiation Protection. Science, Medicine and Technology in Society, 1896–1935" (Ph.D. diss., Princeton University, 1977). On the changing public perception of radiation, see Spencer R. Weart, *Nuclear Fear. A History of Images* (Cambridge, Mass., 1988).

30. On the comparison of the Nuclear Age with the Industrial Revolution, see a paper from Schulten in "Arbeitskreis IV/2 der Deutschen Atomkommission," minutes dated February 22, 1957, Bundesarchiv Koblenz B 138/3413. On the question of safety regulation in relation to public opinion, see "Arbeitskreis IV der Deutschen Atomkommission," minutes dated June 3, 1957, Bundesarchiv Koblenz B 138/566. Radkau (n. 20 above), pp. 392–98, points out that there was a discrepancy between safety rhetoric and specific safety regulations at the beginning of the Nuclear Age in Germany.

31. See, for example, *Strahlentherapie* 32 (1929): 606–11; *Strahlentherapie* 43 (1932): 796–800. As an example of post-war regulations see "Regeln für den Strahlenschutz" [SiB 57/2, Forschungszentrum Karlsruhe. Technik und Umwelt. Hauptabteilung Sicherheit].

32. See, for example, an instrument in the collections of the Deutsches Museum: "Graetz–Dosisleistungsmesser X-50 mit Sonde," Deutsches Museum, Inv. No. 89/466.

33. "Strahlenschutzregelung für das Kernforschungszentrum Karlsruhe," dated March 16, 1961, Generallandesarchiv Karlsruhe 69–599.

34. Paper from Schulten in "Arbeitskreis IV/2 der Deutschen Atomkommission," minutes dated February 22, 1957, Bundesarchiv Koblenz B 138/3413.599.

35. Letter to the Atomic Minister, Balke, dated December 8, 1958, Bundesarchiv Koblenz B 138/571.

36. On the spatial layout of modern high-energy physics laboratories, see Sharon Traweek, *Beamtimes and Lifetimes. The World of High Energy Physics* (Cambridge, Mass., 1988), pp. 18–45; Francoise Zonabend, *The Nuclear Peninsular* (Cambridge, 1993).

37. *Mitteilungsblätter Strahlungsmeßgeräte* (Frieseke & Höpfner, Erlangen) 3 (1960): 13–14.

38. Rajewsky, "Total-Body Radioactivity" (n. 15 above), pp. 18–19. Paper of Straimer in "Fachkommission IV der Deutschen Atomkommission," constituent session, September 13, 1956, Bundesarchiv Koblenz B 138/566. Paper of Atomic Minister Balke, presented in Düsseldorf on November 15, 1957, Generallandesarchiv Karlsruhe 69–150; see also Radkau (n. 20 above), pp. 350–52.

39. Radkau (n. 20 above), pp. 350–52, argued that the tolerance dose did not become a target of American opposition to the nuclear industries until the late 1960s, while the issue has never become a major cause for conflict in Germany. Peter Lundgreen has drawn my attention to the significance of threshold values for the handling of radiation risks.

40. "Jeder Schadensfall ist Beweis schlechter Leitung des Betriebs und mangelnder Führung im Betrieb," Balke (n. 38 above).

41. Directory of authorities for radiation measurements, Bundesarchiv Koblenz B 138/372.

42. The monitoring system of the reactor in Karlsruhe is described in Generallandesarchiv Karlsruhe 69–322.

43. *Strahlungsmeßgerät FH 49. Beschreibung und Betriebsanleitung*, Fa. Eberline Instruments Erlangen, Archiv Frieseke & Hoepfner.

44. "Jahressitzung der Schutzkommission der DFG," dated April 2, 1956, Bundesarchiv Koblenz, B 106/17176; "Übersicht über die Arbeiten des Ausschusses 14 'Radioaktive Niederschläge' der Schutzkommission," Bundesarchiv Koblenz B 106/17177.

45. *Abendzeitung München*, August 20, 1957.

46. Letter to the Ministry of the Interior dated November 12, 1956, Bundesarchiv Koblenz B 106/17162.

47. Meeting at the Ministry of the Interior, April 14, 1955; correspondence between Gentner, Sittkus and Riezler, dated October 26, 1955, Bundesarchiv Koblenz B 106/17162.

48. "Bericht über die Neuerungen auf dem Gebiet der Strahlungsmeßtechnik," February 20, 1957, Bundesarchiv Koblenz B 138/3420.

49. On a classification of radiation measuring instruments and the corresponding strategies for civil defence, see "Ausschuß 2 der Schutzkommission der DFG," minutes dated December 8, 1952 and February 2, 1953, Bundesarchiv Koblenz B 106/17176. See also Wolfgang Riezler (Hg.), *Wissenschaftliche Fragen des zivilen Bevölkerungsschutzes mit besonderer Berücksichtigung der Strahlungsgefährung [Schriftenreihe über zivilen Luftschutz Heft 11]* (Koblenz, 1958).

50. Robert G. Jaeger, *Strahlennachweis- und -meßgeräte [Schriftenreihe über den zivilen Luftschutz Heft 6]* (Koblenz, 1956), p. 28.

51. See, for example, recommendations of Otto Haxel in "Ausschuß 3 der Schutzkommission der DFG," minutes dated October 23, 1952, Bundesarchiv Koblenz B 106/17176. Mary Douglas has provided a framework for the analysis of institutions in charge of risk management. The institutional regulation of hazards is of crucial importance for radiation protection in civil defence, in the workplace and in day-to-day life. For the general argument, see Mary Douglas, *How Institutions Think* (London, 1987) and *Risk Acceptability According to the Social Sciences* (London, 1986).

52. "Ausschuß 2 der Schutzkommission der DFG," minutes dated December 8, 1952, Bundesarchiv Koblenz B 106/17176.

53. Bundesarchiv Koblenz B 106/54498.

54. See, for example, *Spiegel* 5 (May 23, 1951): 24.

55. "Fachkommission IV der Deutschen Atomkommission," constituent session, September 13, 1956, Bundesarchiv Koblenz B 138/566. On public opinion about nuclear energy see Ilona Stölken-Fitschen, *Atombombe und Geistesgeschichte. Eine Studie der fünfziger Jahre aus deutscher Sicht [Nomos-Universitätsschriften / Kulturwissenschaft Bd.3]* (Baden-Baden, 1995) and Matthias Jung, *Öffentlichkeit und Sprachwandel. Zur Geschichte des Diskurses über die Atomenergie* (Opladen, 1994).

56. Johannes Thyssen, "Philosophische Probleme am Anfang des Atomzeitalters," 1958, Bundesarchiv Koblenz B 138/264.

57. "Denn die Bevölkerung der Bundesrepublik muß daran gewöhnt werden, daß es Strahlengefahren gibt, soll andererseits aber auch wissen, daß Maßnahmen dagegen von Amts wegen getroffen werden." Internal note of the Ministry of Agriculture, November 24, 1960, Bundesarchiv Koblenz B 116/14778.

58. Generallandesarchiv Karlsruhe 69–322.

59. Generallandesarchiv Karlsruhe 69–162; 69–351; 69–547.

60. Correspondence of Ernst Georg Miller, January 4, 1965, Bundesarchiv Koblenz B 106/54502.

61. Volks-Geiger counter "AGFA Ray-O-Mat," 1959, Deutsches Museum, Inv. Nr. 74647.

62. Note dated October 19, 1961, Bundesarchiv Koblenz B 106/54502.

63. "Erst flotte Tanzmusik – dann tickt der Geigerzähler. Das Radio im Taschenformat zugleich Meßgerät für Radioaktivität. Erfindung eines gebürtigen Augsburgers," *Augsburger Allgemeine*, March 30, 1962, Bundesarchiv Koblenz B 106/54502.

64. *Frankfurter Allgemeine Zeitung* (June 28, 1962), Generallandesarchiv Karlsruhe 69–904.

65. "Der Einzelne hat keinerlei Möglichkeit, die tatsächliche Gefahr einer radioaktiven Verseuchung zu beurteilen. Daran ändert auch ein Volksgeigerzähler nichts," note dated August 9, 1962, Generallandesarchiv Karlsruhe 69–904.

66. "Schutzkommission der DFG," meeting on May 30, 1959, Bundesarchiv Koblenz B 106/1778.

67. "Sobald man eine Gefahr fassen kann, ist ihre Gefährlichkeit ja schon beseitigt," *Durlacher Tagblatt*, November 27, 1956, Generallandesarchiv Karlsruhe 69–547.

Patricia Peck Gossel

Packaging the Pill

Doctors have long been plagued with patients who failed to take their medicine. Only recently have packages for prescription drugs been designed to help patients remember. The "Dialpak",[1] issued in 1963 with the oral contraceptive Ortho-Novum, appears to have been the first "compliance package" for a prescription drug – one that is intended to help the patient comply with the doctor's orders. This distinctive package and the social notoriety of the birth control pill ("the Pill") have made it the most readily recognised prescription drug on the market. Since G. D. Searle & Co. introduced the first oral contraceptive in 1960, the Pill's package has become familiar to both men and women from its depiction on the covers of news-stand magazines and popular books,[2] although a single tablet of an oral contraceptive, if separated from its container, could be recognised only by an experienced pharmacist.

Not surprisingly, the revolution in drug packaging heralded by the Dialpak has been overlooked in the midst of other revolutions associated with the Pill. Yet design changes in the package had a significant pharmacological effect – the number of hormone-containing pills in each prescription was increased. This unexpected result from what seems a rather inconsequential accessory to a complex medical technology will be used to illustrate the important part that consumer concerns, product presentation and patent issues play in establishing pharmaceutical regimens.

Historians who have studied the oral contraceptive have concentrated on its scientific development and progress through drug approval legislation, the public furore over its side-effects, and its role in the sexual and social revolutions of the 1960s and 1970s. Little has been said about the Pill's manufacture and production, and its package has gone unnoticed in histories of the Pill; in fact, little has been written on the history of drug packaging. The cultural context that historians have provided for the Pill has been that of the society at large or women as a group. Recently, Elizabeth Watkins has shown how the Pill changed women's relationships with their physicians. Lara Marks' studies of the clinical trials of the oral contraceptive have examined the problem of patient compliance with research protocols.[3] The history of the compliance packaging for the Pill provides another example of the way issues unrelated to the medical science of chemical contraception affected women's daily experience with the Pill and also contributed to medical opinion of women in the 1960s.

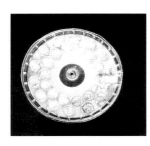

Figure 1. David P. Wagner's pill dispenser prototype is made of three round plastic plates held by a snap fastener. The bottom plate has the day-of-the-week pattern, the middle plate holds twenty wooden "pills" in a pattern that rotates to match the day pill-taking begins, a single hole in the top plate is moved over the pill to dispense it. As each pill is dispensed, the day of the week is revealed as a reminder that the pill was taken.

This history of the compliance packaging for the Pill is based on prototypes of the first container designed to hold the oral contraceptive, and on a study of the oral contraceptive and advertising in the collections of the Division of Science, Medicine and Society at the Smithsonian's National Museum of American History. The packaging prototypes came to the Smithsonian's collections as the result of a case study of the birth control pill in the Museum's *Science in American Life* exhibit, which opened in April 1994. Dr Celso-Ramón García, who had directed some of the first clinical trials of oral contraceptives, saw the large display of birth control pills in the exhibit and put me in touch with the inventor of the Pill package. The following year, its inventor, David P. Wagner of Geneva, Illinois, donated his prototypes and a small but fascinating collection that includes his design drawings, patent, correspondence, legal documents, and examples of oral contraceptive packages that either did or did not fall within the claims of his patent.[4] The examination of these packages and advertisements was central to this study.

***

David P. Wagner invented his dispenser to help his wife remember to take her Pill. Doris Wagner began taking the Pill after their fourth child, Jane, was born on November 14, 1961, and the Wagners decided that their family was complete. The only oral contraceptive on the market in 1961 was Enovid, from G. D. Searle & Co. Prescriptions for Enovid were dispensed as tablets in a small brown bottle. Instructions for taking the Pill seemed straightforward: Doris was to take the first tablet on the fifth day after beginning menstruation, continue with one tablet every day for 20 days, and then stop; she would begin menstruating in two to three days, and on the fifth day of menstruation she was to start another 20-day cycle of tablets. The 20-pill regimen originated in the 1940s, when hormones were first used to treat menstrual problems. It was selected for the oral contraceptive clinical trials so that the hormonally controlled cycle would conform to the average or "normal" 28-day menstrual cycle and would encourage women to view the method as "natural."[5]

David Wagner recalled, "there was a lot of room for error in whether 'the Pill' was actually taken on a given day." He said, "I found that I was just as concerned as Doris was in whether she had taken her pill or not. I was constantly asking her whether she had taken 'the Pill' and this led to some irritation and a marital row or two."[6] To resolve their frustrations, Wagner listed the days of the week on a piece of paper, put the paper on the dresser in their bedroom, and placed one pill over each day. When Doris removed a pill, the day of the week would be revealed and they could both tell, at a glance, whether she had taken her pill. "This did wonders for our relationship. It lasted for about two or three weeks until something fell and scattered the pills and the paper all over the floor."[7] Still, he liked the

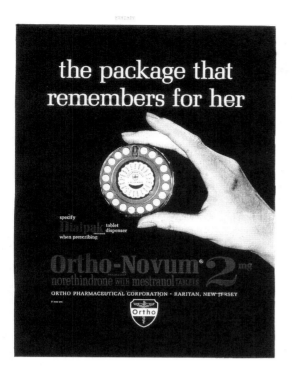

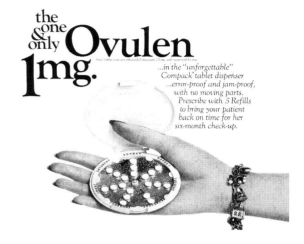

Figure 3. G. D. Searle & Co.'s Compack used a foil blister pack refill that had to be oriented so the black arrow pointed to the day menstrual flow began. The first pill to be taken was marked by a black circle.

Figure 2. This 1964 Ortho-Novum advertisement shows the first Dialpak dispenser for the oral contraceptive.

basic idea, but he needed some kind of container to keep the pills oriented to the day of the week, yet prevent them from spilling, even if his wife carried them in her purse. He started "noodling around," and sketched variations of such a pill box.

David Wagner was more than a clever spouse: he was educated to take a technological approach to problem solving. He worked as a product engineer developing new fasteners for Illinois Tool Works, and he already held one patent at the time he invented his dispenser. He recalled:

At this point, I felt I had a pretty good idea, but if I was going to interest anyone in it, I felt I needed several models. So, with just a 1/4" electric drill, a fly cutter to be used in the drill, paper, a saw, a staple, pencil, double-faced transparent tape, several drill bits, a snap fastener that I took off of a child's toy, and several flat, clear sheets of either acrylic or polycarbonate plastic, I fashioned the first pill box for packaging birth control pills. My model is dated 5-15-62. I simulated the pill by sawing thin slices from a wooden dowel rod.[8] (*see* Figure 1)

Wagner applied to patent his invention on July 27, 1962, with the help of a friend who was a patent attorney. Soon afterwards, he paid a visit to the Director of Advertising for G. D. Searle & Co. He said that Searle "felt basically my pill box was a good idea, but at that particular time they were preoccupied with establishing a market and overcoming some adverse publicity."[9] He had had the misfortune to approach Searle after it became known that some women taking Enovid had died from blood clots.[10]

Wagner had read that Ortho Pharmaceutical also was working on a birth control pill, and he sent them one of his models in the autumn of 1962. A few months later, on February 1, 1963, Ortho placed on the market its first oral contraceptive, Ortho-Novum, in an attractive dispenser called the "Dialpak." Ortho advertised the Dialpak (*see* Figure 2) prominently, to distinguish its product from the competition. It appeared to Wagner that their design resembled the claims of his patent. As soon as Wagner was issued his patent – on August 4, 1964, a year and a half after the Dialpak appeared on the market – he and his lawyer moved to enforce it. In December 1964 he received his first income from the invention – a cheque from Ortho for $10,000, in return for signing an agreement not to sue them.[11]

Wagner made use of Ortho's success to encourage Searle to re-examine his invention, even before he was awarded his patent. Ortho's Dialpak had demonstrated the marketing value of his idea and had shown that it could be manufactured "for pennies" as a disposable container. Wagner argued to Searle that his version of the dispenser was easier to understand and operate than the Dialpak, and it would help Searle protect its market share.[12] Searle again rejected his dispenser, on the grounds that they did not feel the need for promotional devices.[13] Searle's view of unique packaging as an advertising gimmick is hardly surprising. Drug companies were known in the design community for their "ingrained cautiousness" and the "numbing sameness" of their packaging – a conservatism required, in part, by the need to conform to federal regulations.[14] Yet, when Searle introduced its new, lower dose, Enovid-E in 1964, that, too, came in a special memory dispenser (*see* Figure 3). In 1966, Searle agreed to pay Wagner royalties on the packages for two of their oral contraceptives, Enovid-E and 1 mg Ovulen.[15]

Over the years, Wagner received about $130,000 after legal fees, from his initial $30 investment in materials. The patent earned $0.0020–0.0025 per dispenser, according to the legal documents that he signed with Ortho and Searle. He was also paid by Upjohn, the Canadian subsidiary of Organon, Inc., Eli Lilly, and Mead Johnson.[16] Eventually, Wagner tired of fighting for his royalties and sold Ortho Pharmaceutical an undivided half interest in his patent in 1973. It was his last licence for use of the patent.

***

The origin of the compliance dispenser as an inspiration from the spouse of a patient, rather than from the pharmaceutical company that developed and marketed the product, challenges assumptions about where to look for the source of innovation. It also raises the question of whether pharmaceutical companies ever had any interest in packages designed to aid patient memory. Surely, such packaging might have appealed to a company's proprietary interests? With a product such as the birth control pill, women who failed to take oral contraceptives correctly and became pregnant were likely to lose confidence in oral contraceptives, and lost confidence could be expected to damage sales. As Searle initially dismissed Wagner's invention, just how unique was his dispenser as a form of pharmaceutical packaging?

Means of reassuring patients that they have taken their medication or reminding them that it's time for another dose have existed for a long time. Nineteenth-century medical spoons in the Smithsonian collections have handles with dial reminders for the convenience of either the patient or the care-giver.[17] A search of the US Patent Office records provided a few other examples, such as a tray patented by Mary C. Mottayaw of Mansfield, Ohio in 1929 that allowed an entire day's medicines to be laid out correctly, and provided a place for setting a timepiece.[18] The Patent Office has surprisingly few examples of similar pill-taking aids until the 1950s, and none are presented as packaging for prescription drugs.

Traditionally, prescription-drug packaging has been designed to protect the integrity of the product while it is in transit from the factory. Pharmacists routinely have dispensed prescription drugs into drab, nearly identical bottles or vials, from larger bottles provided by the drug company. Innovations such as child-proof caps and tamper-proof packages came from consumer-stimulated regulations intended to protect children from accidental poisoning or to prevent malicious tampering with non-prescription drugs, as in the recent Tylenol scare.[19] Unit-dose packages, in which each dose is separately packaged, emerged in the 1960s in hospital pharmacies to control errors made when nurses dispensed medicines to inpatients on the wards.[20]

The advent of plastics brought new flexibility to package design, but, until the 1960s, few drug companies adopted plastics for prescription-drug packaging. New materials, such as high-density polyethylene, that could replace glass bottles without costly changes in assembly-line filling equipment were adopted primarily because they cut shipping costs, reduced space requirements and did not break in transit. Some more elaborate plastic dispensers for non-prescription drugs are known from the 1950s: Squibb introduced its "Trak-pak" in 1954 to promote aspirin and used it again in 1962 for saccharine, and vitamins such as Squibb's Vigran and cold medications such as Schering's Coricidin were also packaged in dispensers that combined polystyrene and high-density polyethylene. Although none of these designs incorporated memory aids, consumers liked the convenience, and felt that they acquired more for their money when they received a dispenser.[21] The kind of consumer manipulation that we associate with package designs intended both to advertise and to sell has been conspicuously absent from pharmaceutical products available only by prescription.[22]

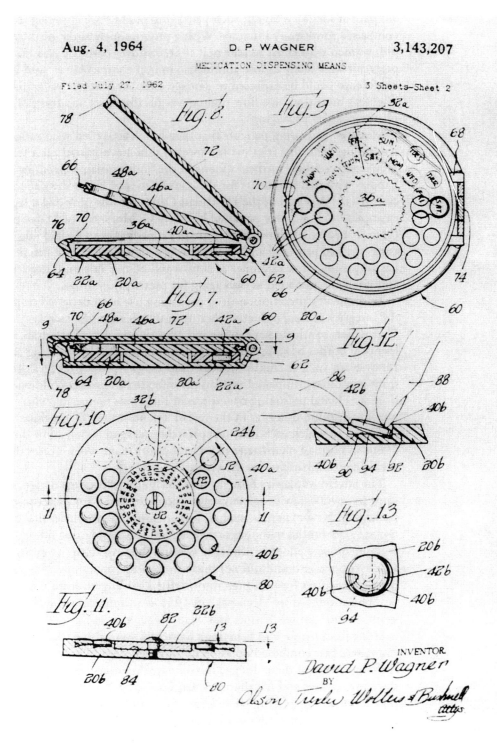

Figure 4. An illustration of the compact version of David P. Wagner's pill dispenser from US Patent # 3,143,207.

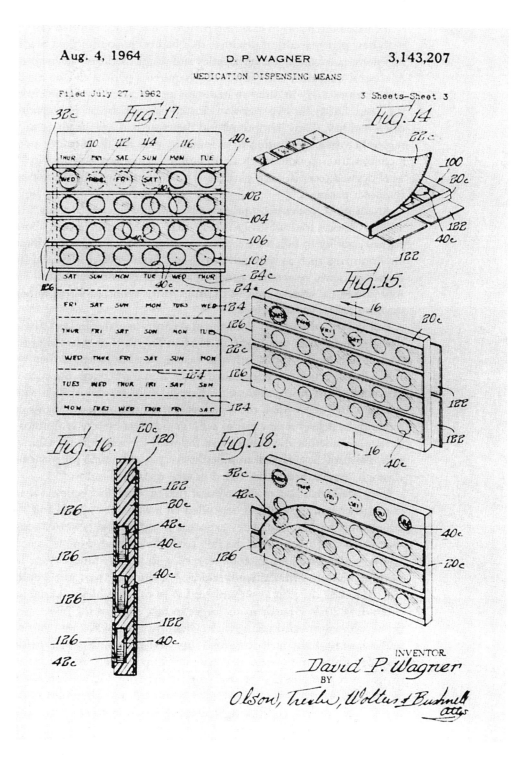

Figure 5. An illustration of a less costly rectangular version of David P. Wagner's pill dispenser from US Patent # 3,143,207. A sheet of paper is pulled through until the starting day is oriented to the first place on the top row (Fig. 17 Wednesday). The first pill, to be taken on the fifth day, is shown covering Sunday (Fig. 17).

Increased attention to ensuring patient compliance came in the 1950s with new pharmaceutical products that had more complicated medical regimens, particularly the antibiotics and drugs used to treat hypertension. Successful treatment with antibiotics required a patient to take medicine several times a day in order to maintain an effective blood concentration of the drug. Drugs for hypertension created concern, because the patients often had few, if any, symptoms and therefore had less incentive to remember their medication than someone who felt ill. Memory aids such as a combination pocket-watch alarm and pill container, patented in 1960, were devised to assist such patients. The drugs themselves did not come in reminder packages.[23]

Attention to patient compliance also emerged in clinical trials during the 1950s. Clinical trials of drugs initially had raised little concern about a patient's ability to follow directions, as most were conducted in monitored environments such as hospitals or prisons. Even in field trials with freely mobile patients, researchers generally determined compliance by monitoring the concentrations of drugs in the blood or urine, rather than devising tactics to aid memory.[24]

Compliance difficulties with the oral contraceptive emerged first during the large field trials that began in 1956 in Puerto Rico, Los Angeles, Mexico and Haiti. Applicants who were assessed as having difficulty in following directions were excluded at the initial interview. Social workers provided careful instruction and follow-up visits for the women who were enrolled. In Puerto Rico, the social worker visited the participants once a month to deliver a new vial of pills, gather data on any symptoms and determine whether the women had followed the schedule for taking the pills. Nevertheless, a small number in every trial became pregnant because, through "carelessness", they failed to take their medication.[25]

Lara Marks has shown that clinical trial investigators believed that compliance with procedures depended on a woman's cultural and educational background. They expected wealthier and better-educated women to continue to take the Pill, but believed that those who needed it most – deprived and illiterate women with large families – were less likely to comply with daily pill-taking. For the most part, the women in the trials took the pills as prescribed, but in one troublesome trial in Haiti, more than 20% of participants forgot to take some of the pills. Some women stopped taking them when their husbands were out of town, and others took them all at once. Many of these women could neither read nor count, so the calendars supplied as reminders were of little help. To enhance compliance, the trial team tried giving the women rosary beads, with instructions to move one bead each day when they took a pill. Nevertheless, confusion persisted. Some women wore the beads instead, thinking that the rosary beads alone protected them against pregnancy. Marks notes that "clearly much depended not only on the educational background of women, but also on individual motivation

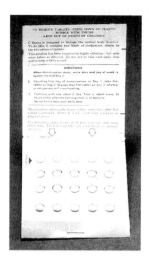

Figure 6. C-Quens, the first sequential oral contraceptive in the USA was distributed by Eli Lilly. It contained two different formulations that had to be taken in sequence. The paper package requested the woman write down the date and day menstruation started to keep track of the regimen.

in the success of following instructions, as well as the skill of the instructor."[26]

Despite such difficulties, common in the clinical trials, the official reports mention the problems with compliance primarily to explain that pregnancies among the trial patients could not be attributed to technical failure of the oral contraceptive. As long as all pregnancies among trial participants could be dismissed as the result of a deliberate choice to become pregnant or the result of a woman's failure to follow instructions, the contraceptive could be deemed 100% successful. Researchers acknowledged that compliance was a problem, but considered it an issue primarily for international population planners who worked with poor, illiterate women.[27] The physicians' conclusions that the method was highly popular and their belief that most women were highly motivated to follow the instructions gave them little reason to encourage G. D. Searle & Company to include memory devices with the Pill.

Once Ortho introduced the Dialpak however, every new birth control pill on the market came with some kind of memory aid. Two primary features determined whether a package fell under the claims of Wagner's patent: (1) the pills were retained in a pattern and (2) they could be adjusted in relation to an element having day-of-the-week identification (*see* Figures 4 and 5). Wagner found that the pharmaceutical companies were naturally reluctant to pay royalties to "outside" inventors, and either argued strongly that their packages did not infringe his patent, or worked to develop a dispensing device that would not infringe the patent.[28] As drug companies introduced new oral contraceptives to the market, they distinguished their products from their competition both through changes in the pill formulation and through changes in the packaging.

Packages that included reminders for the 20-day regimen invariably required some mechanical means of altering the date in relation to the tablet, as the regimen did not fit neatly into the seven-day week. As a result, they invariably fell under the claims of Wagner's patent. The package for Eli Lilly's C-Quens, the first sequential Pill on the American market, introduced in 1965, illustrates the difficulty (*see* Figure 6). With sequential pills, it was important that the pills be taken in the correct order. C-Quens maintained the 20-day regimen, but gave 15 days of estrogen, followed by five days of an estrogen/progestogen combination, arranging the pills in four rows of five tablets. The package superficially resembled a calendar, but, other than a place to note the date on which the first pill was taken, it offered the taker no help in remembering if she missed a day.[29]

The desire to avoid conflict with Wagner's patent resulted in design changes that altered the pill-taking regimen. Searle first introduced Ovulen in an adjustable compact identical to the Enovid-E container. The package for Searle's 1-mg oral contraceptive, Ovulen, changed after they agreed to pay royalties to Wagner. Searle reissued the drug as Ovulen-21, in a rectangular compact which added an additional pill to the cycle as a means

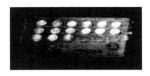

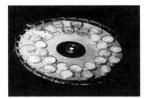

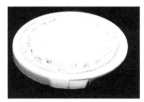

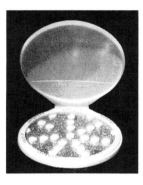

Figure 7. G. D. Searle and Co.'s oral contraceptives are shown with David P. Wagner's prototype (top and second from top). Enovid-E 20 (third) and Ovulen-20 (bottom) had features covered by Wagner's patent.

to avoid adjusting the date – a critical element in Wagner's patent (*see* Figures 7 and 8). Their advertising copy alerted doctors to the change: "Ovulen-21, works the way a woman thinks by weekdays … not 'cycle days.' Ovulen-21 lets her remember her natural way. Once established, her starting day is always the same day of the week … because it is fixed at three weeks on – one week off and is independent of withdrawal flow."[30] The 21-day regimen proved so popular that Ortho brought out their 2-mg pill in a 21-day form, despite retaining their distinctive Dialpak dispenser.[31]

Organon Laboratories in the UK created a 22-tablet regimen for their 2.5-mg oral contraceptive, Lyndiol. They reasoned, as their advertising flyers indicate, that "maximum patient reliability" is ensured when "each course of tablets always begins and ends on the same fixed day of the week … Thus, if the "last" tablet is taken on a Friday evening, then the first tablet from the next pack is taken on the next Friday evening."[32] Women throughout the world who used Organon oral contraceptives had their menstrual cycles adjusted to this new regimen. Geigy of Germany also used the 22-tablet regimen for their 2-mg birth control pill, Yermonil.[33]

The calendar pack made it evident that, by adding placebos, women could take a pill every day. Oracon, a sequential birth control pill introduced by Mead Johnson in 1965, was available in both a 21-day and a 28-day version.[34] The ease of giving instructions for taking the 28-day Pill made that version popular with medical personnel. The simplicity of the 28-day regimen also ensured that the new sequential pills would be taken in the correct order. Theoretically, women could start to take their pills any day of the week, but they especially liked the "Sunday start," as it duplicated the calendar and resulted in "period-free weekends."[35]

Changes in pill formulation and package design followed the move to the 28-day regimen. The desire that every pill should do something encouraged Parke–Davis to add iron compounds to the seven placebos in 1-mg Norlestrin Fe, as a nutritional supplement to compensate for mineral loss during menstrual bleeding.[36] Because women now took a pill every day, many companies abandoned the calendar format, simply adding graphic arrows to a rectangular arrangement of pills in a blister pack to ensure that the user took the pills in the proper sequence.[37] In some cases the pill count per package also varied, as illustrated by examples of 35-tablet and 42-tablet packages.[38]

Package designs for the oral contraceptive were developed that elicited other medically beneficial behavioural changes. One design incorporated a dial to remind a woman to self-examine her breasts for tumours at the optimum time of her cycle, between days seven and twelve.[39] Recently, a randomised clinical trial found that even simple prompts resulted in higher rates of self-examination of the breasts. The package design used for the clinical trial simply added the statement, "best time for Breast Self Exam – 7 days after period end" beneath the first row of pills on a calendar pack.[40]

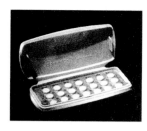

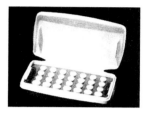

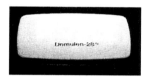

Figure 8. Searle's Enovid-E 21 (top) Ovulen-28 (middle) and Demulen-28 (bottom), all in rectangular compacts, used a 21-day cycle, required no orientation to the day of the week, and were not covered by Wagner's patent.

Aesthetic changes in birth control pill packages reflected societal norms, especially the desire to keep birth control discrete. David Wagner, in his patent, claimed his Pill dispenser would fit into a case "indistinguishable" from a lady's cosmetic "compact," so that it could be carried among her personal effects or in her purse, "without giving a visible clew [sic] as to matters which are of no concern to others."[41] Plastic Pill "compacts" from the 1960s were produced in pastel colours with cameo and floral designs pressed into their surfaces. By the 1980s, the cases were as likely to look like wallets or be designed to resemble credit cards.

Although packaging changes made it easier for women to remember to take the birth control pill, daily pill-taking remained one of the disadvantages of oral contraceptives (*see* Figure 9). A 1965 study of 5,600 women cited psychological difficulties such as worry about forgetting to take the Pill every morning, and a general dislike of taking a pill every day, among the reasons women switched to other methods of contraception.[42] For women who missed a Pill, the dispenser reminded them that they might face an unwanted pregnancy, and it seemed to them like "contraceptive roulette," according to *Newsweek*.[43] One study gave Pill users psychological tests and identified a range of "pill forgetters' defects" such as the inability to assume responsibility, control impulses or appreciate long-range goals.[44]

Women's "forgetfulness" problem became a common theme of oral-contraceptive advertising in medical journals in the late 1960s, even when the package design was not featured prominently. These advertisements, directed at physicians, repeated the paternalistic view of the doctor–patient relationship common at the time and sometimes presented women as scatter-brained, incompetent and in need of guidance. At the same time, by encouraging doctors to take a more active role in educating the patient, the advertisements hinted that doctors had previously provided poor instructions. Organon depicted a woman who was "newly wed …, working still …, madly busy …, mind awhirl," and urged doctors to "Protect the new patient from her own forgetfulness."[45] The British Drug Houses of Canada, in promoting their new 28-day sequential oral contraceptive, assured doctors that "Now you can give her a 'pill' that really counts for her."[46]

Gynecology textbooks and consumer manuals offered helpful suggestions for overcoming the problem of "forgetfulness."[47] For the most part, these seem to be obvious solutions: keep your pills next to your toothbrush, next to the kitchen range, or take them with a particular meal. A Philadelphia women's health clinic recommended that women take their Pill when they heard the theme music for the 11 o'clock news.[48] Most of their clients listened to the news, and taking the Pill just before bedtime had the double advantage that women who became dizzy or nauseous as a result of taking it slept through the discomfort. In 1993, Organon incorporated this genre of reminder into their "Remember Me Compliance Kit" for Desogen.

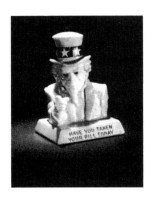

Figure 9. This Uncle Sam figurine asks "Have you taken your pill today?" It dates from 1969 protests over the distribution of oral contraceptives through US government-funded health clinics.

The package of birth control pills was presented in a box with a toothbrush, a small bar of soap, a "Remember Me" sticker for the bathroom mirror and the slogan "Brush your teeth, wash your face, take your pill ... once a day, everyday, at the same time."[49] As an incentive to persuade doctors to prescribe their products, Organon supplied doctors with these complimentary kits to initiate their new oral-contraceptive patients. That so many pharmaceutical company advertisements and gynecology manuals addressed the "forgetfulness" problem, and couples such as the Wagners actively sought methods to keep track of taking the Pill, suggests how complex it was to follow the on-again, off-again 20-tablet cycle, and what an important contribution the compliance package made.

***

Norplant, representing another example of changes made to a chemical contraceptive to overcome compliance problems, also illustrates the importance of attention to the design and production of medical technologies, and their potential medical and social effects. The Population Council sponsored new research on a chemical contraceptive for international population control that aimed to eliminate altogether the problem of forgetfulness, at the time when pharmaceutical companies were changing package designs to overcome Wagner's patent. This, too, involved an element of packaging – in this case, a unique drug capsule. In 1964, the Population Council's Center for Biomedical Research demonstrated that hormones could be released from silicone rubber capsules implanted in the body. By 1975, clinical trials of a chemical contraceptive in a six-capsule "silastic drug delivery system" implanted under the skin on the inside of a woman's upper arm were under way in several countries. The contraceptive was named Norplant by its manufacturer, Wyeth-Ayerst, and was first approved for use in Finland in 1983. By the mid 1990s, 15 countries had approved it for marketing.[50] In 1983, levonorgestrel, the pharmaceutical agent used in Norplant, had already been on the market for some years, in the progestin-only mini-pill and in several of the widely used combination Pills.

Clearly, a drug-delivery system represents a different category of compliance packaging than the date-adjustable dispenser. In this case, the dosage form and the container have, in a sense, merged. Previous attempts to extend the effects of drugs had depended on the solubility of a medication or its coating, but the entire product was consumed by the patient. A series of innovations in the 1970s introduced the infusion pump used in intensive care units, transdermal patches, and osmotic systems that both contained and protected a drug while it was released in a controlled way over long periods of time.[51] In the case of Norplant, the silastic tubes filled with powdered levonorgestrel remained under the skin of the woman's arm until the spent container/drug-delivery device was removed by her doctor, five years later.

Dependence on the medical establishment for prescriptions has made oral contraceptives the bane of the women's self-help medical movement ever since the Pill was introduced.[52] Unlike barrier devices or contraceptive foams and jellies, over which a woman and her partner had complete control, the birth control pill required women to obtain an annual or semi-annual prescription from a physician or a health clinic. Norplant was a boon for women who wanted long-term contraception and found it difficult to remember a daily pill. However, its need to be medically removed made women even more dependent on their medical providers when making decisions about reproduction than did the Pill, which a woman could stop taking whenever she wished.

More seriously, because of its package/drug-delivery system, Norplant could be used to enforce compliance coercively. In the USA, the desire to implement such uses accompanied Norplant from the day it was approved, December 10, 1990.[53] Newspaper columnist Ellen Goodman reported that, the first day Norplant was announced, a caller to a radio talk-show proclaimed that every girl should have Norplant stuck in her arm at puberty. The next day, the *Philadelphia Inquirer* published an editorial urging readers to "think about" Norplant as a tool in the fight against black poverty.[54] A California judge ordered a woman, who was guilty of child abuse, to have Norplant inserted as part of a plea bargain.[55] Legislatures in 11 states proposed bills (although they passed none of them) to offer financial incentives to women receiving welfare, to encourage them to use Norplant.[56] Federal Medicaid paid for the insertion of the implants, but states control Medicaid distribution, and in South Dakota, for example, Medicaid would not pay for the removal of Norplant in the absence of a medical reason for doing so.[57] Such incidents, in the USA and in other countries, have raised alarms about the potential for misuse of Norplant.[58] For the purposes of this paper, the example is provided in order to emphasise that it was not the hormone in Norplant, but rather its form of *packaging*, that made this contraceptive so easily subject to coercive use.

***

Auxiliary technologies such as the pharmaceutical package are usually overlooked, but, as the examples of the compliance package and Norplant illustrate, they have both medical and social repercussions. This account argues for the usefulness of studying the artefacts themselves. Examination of the diverse packages for birth control pills in the collections of the National Museum of American History revealed that the number of pills in a package varied from one brand of oral contraceptive to another. Who would have guessed that this difference originated to help women remember to take their pill?

Since the introduction of the Dialpak, compliance packages have become far more common. Drugs with unusual dosage schedules are now likely to come from the pharmaceutical manufacturer in "unit-of-use" compliance packages designed to let the patient know at a glance when to take the pills each day – packages that also eliminate the need for the doctor or pharmacist to explain complicated schedules. Now, clinical trials can use bottle caps with microelectronic devices that record the time and date when the patient removes the lid to take a pill.[59] Patient compliance as a health-care issue has gained greater salience in association with increasing health-care costs, aging patients who take multiple medications, and the increase in prominence of chronic diseases associated with lifestyle.

David Wagner started a quiet revolution in package design for prescription drugs, which one would have expected either to come from a pharmaceutical or packaging company, or to have been requested by physicians prescribing oral contraceptives. Rarely are patients or their families considered as sources of innovation and change in medical technologies. Histories of medical technologies, even when they take into consideration the concerns of the patient, portray patients as passive objects to which medical technologies are applied. Patients may request or refuse technical procedures, but the source of change or innovation in a technology invariably is assumed to reside in a dialogue between the doctor, the institution and the inventor or engineer.[60] The example of the Pill package challenges easy assumptions about sources of change in medical technology and speaks for the importance of considering the whole of a technology when evaluating its medical and social effects.

Notes

1. A note on terminology: Dialpak is a registered trademark of the Ortho Pharmaceutical Company. When capitalised, "Pill" has come, through common parlance, to designate the birth control pill or the oral contraceptive and it will be so used here.
2. See, for example, the cover of *Maclean's*, April 17, 1978, and the jacket cover of Robert W. Kistner, *The Pill; Facts and Fallacies About Today's Oral Contraceptives* (New York, 1968).
3. General histories of the oral contraceptive include James Reed, *From Private Vice to Public Virtue* (New York, 1978), pp. 309–66; Angus McLaren, *A History of Contraception From Antiquity to the Present Day* (London, 1990), pp. 239–67; A. D. G. Gunn, *Oral Contraception in Perspective* (Carnforth, Lancs, UK, 1987); William H. Robertson, *An Illustrated History of Contraception* (Carnforth, Lancs, UK, 1990), pp. 121–38; and Bernard Asbell, *The Pill: A Biography of the Drug that Changed the World* (New York, 1995). Elizabeth Watkins, "On the Pill: How Oral Contraceptives Contributed to Changes in the Practice of Medicine in the Early 1960s," a paper presented at the American Association for the History of Medicine, April 30, 1994, discusses the Pill and its role in making women more assertive in their medical care. Linda Grant, *Sexing the Millenium* (New York, 1994) examines the pill and the sexual revolution. Lara Marks, "'A "Cage" of Ovulating Females': The History of the Early Oral Contraceptive Pill Clinical Trials, 1950–1959," in *Molecularizing Biology and Medicine, 1910s–1970s*, ed. H. Kamminga and S. De Chadarevian (Amsterdam, 1998) is the first historian to look carefully at the research behind the clinical trials. Gena Corea, *The Hidden Malpractice: How American Medicine Mistreats Women* (New York, 1985) understates the extent of the clinical trials to support her argument. FDA historian Suzanne White-Junod examined the basis for approving the Pill in "FDA's Approval of the Contraceptive Pill," a paper presented to the Washington Society for the History of Medicine, January 14, 1993.
4. David P. Wagner Collection, Division of Science, Medicine, and Society, National Museum of American History, Smithsonian Institution, Washington, DC.

5. Lara Marks, "'Andromeda Freed from her Chains': Attitudes Towards Women and the Oral Contraceptive Pill, 1950–1970," in *Women and Medicine*, ed. Anne Hardy and Lawrence Conrad (forthcoming), p. 17; Nelly Oudshoorn, *Beyond the Natural Body* (London, 1994), p. 121.

6. David P. Wagner to Patricia Gossel, January 16, 1995, Wagner Collection.

7. Ibid.

8. Ibid.

9. David P. Wagner to John L. Scott, April 19, 1963, Wagner Collection.

10. G. D. Searle & Co., Press Release, August 9, 1962, Science Service Collection, Smithsonian Institution Archives.

11. Wagner to Gossel (n. 6 above); "Agreement between David P. Wagner and Ortho Pharmaceutical Company," November 25, 1964, Wagner Collection. The first patent for a dial dispenser found with Ortho Pharmaceutical Corporation listed as assignee is US Patent 3,557,747 awarded January 26, 1971.

12. Wagner to Scott (n. 9 above).

13. John L. Scott to David P. Wagner, June 14, 1963, Wagner Collection.

14. "Survey of an Industry 1: Packaging Drugs," *Industrial Design* 10, no. 11 (November 1963): 87–91.

15. David P. Wagner, "Covenant Not to Sue G. D. Searle and Company," August 15, 1966, Wagner Collection.

16. Wagner to Gossel (n. 6 above); "Agreement between Wagner and Ortho" (n. 11 above); "Covenant not to Sue Searle" (n. 15 above).

17. Invalid spoon Pat. no. 51748, Cat. no. M–4303, David J. Pearson, donor, Medical Science Collection, National Museum of American History; invalid spoons and dial reminder, Cat. nos. 1994.243.13, 1994.243.14, 1994.243.33, Dorothy Rainwater, donor, Medical Science Collection. With the American enthusiasm for self-dosing, patents for medical spoons flourished in the 1870s through 1890s, see John S. Haller, "Medical Spoons: A Brief Look at Patents of the 1870s and 1880s," *New York State Journal of Medicine* 93 (1993): 183–88. On the use of medical spoons to calibrate the dose, see George Griffenhagen, "Dose: One Spoonful," *Journal of the American Pharmaceutical Association*, 20 (1959): 202–05.

18. US Patent 1,717,060, "Time Chart," issued to Mary C. Mottayaw, Mansfield, Ohio, June 11, 1929.

19. Very little literature exists on the history of prescription-drug packaging. An important exception is William H. Helfand and David L. Cowen, "Evolution of Pharmaceutical Oral Dosage Forms," *Pharmacy in History* 25 (1983): 3–18. See also, "The Search for Tamper-Proof Packaging: The Protection of Product Integrity," A Pictorial Exhibit, The Pharmacist Institute of New Jersey, 1983; and Aimee Rhum, *Tamper Resistant Packaging: What's Ahead?* (Stamford, CN, 1984).

20. Frost and Sullivan, Inc., *Unit Dose Packaged Pharmaceutical Products in Europe* (New York, 1978), pp. 27–28.

21. "Survey of an Industry" (n. 14 above), pp. 87–91; "New Role for Plastics in Drugs," *Modern Packaging* 37, no. 5 (January 1964): 100–03.

22. Thomas Hine, *The Total Package: The Evolution and Secret Meanings of Boxes, Bottles, Cans, and Tubes* (Boston, 1995) and Stanley Sacharow, *The Package as a Marketing Tool* (Radnor, PA, 1982) also attend to the development of package design.

23. US Patent 2,853,182, "Pocket Chronometer and Pill Container," issued to Harry E. Barnett, Chicago, Ill., September 23, 1958.

24. R. B. Haynes et al., *Compliance in Health Care* (Baltimore, 1979); Susan Jay, Iris F. Litt, and Robert H. Durant, "Compliance with Therapeutic Regimens," *Journal of Adolescent Health Care* 5 (1984): 124–36. See also Daniel A. Hussar, "Patient Compliance," in *Remington's Pharmaceutical Sciences*, 17th ed. (Easton, PA, 1985), pp. 1764–77.

25. Gregory Pincus et al., "Fertility Control with Oral Medication," *American Journal of Obstetrics and Gynecology* 75 (1958): 1343.

26. Marks, "A 'Cage' of Ovulating Females" (n. 3 above), p. 17; Marks, "Andromeda Freed from her Chains" (n. 5 above), pp. 19–20.

27. Edward T. Tyler et al., "An Oral Contraceptive: A Four Year Study of Norethindrone," *Obstetrics and Gynecology* 18 (1961): 367.

28. Wagner to Gossel (n. 6 above).

29. Eli Lilly and Company, "Lilly News," May 5, 1965, Science Service Collection; "C–Quens" oral contraceptive, Cat. no. 82.531.11, Medical Sciences Collection.

30. 1 mg Ovulen advertisement attached to "Covenant Not to Sue Searle" (n. 15 above); "Ovulen-21 Works the Way a Woman Thinks," Searle advertisement, *Virginia Medical Monthly* (August 1968).

31. Ortho trade literature, Syntex Files, Medical Science Collection, National Museum of American History.

32. "In Oral Contraception Lyndiol 2.5 Meets the Case," Organon trade literature, Syntex Files, Medical Science Collection, 1968.

33. Yermonil advertisement, Ciba–Geigy trade literature, Syntex Files, Medical Sciences Collection, July 1975.

34. Oracon oral contraceptive, Cat. no. 81.760.123, Medical Science Collection; Oracon 28 oral contraceptive, Cat. no. 85.475.143, ibid.

35. Greg Juhn, *Understanding the Pill: A Consumer's Guide to Oral Contraceptives* (New York, 1994), p. 31.

36. Parke, Davis and Company, News Release, March 7, 1969, Contraceptive Pills – Various Makers File, Science Service Collection.

37. As an example, see Eugynon ED advertisement, Schering Pty Ltd, *Medical Journal of Australia Advertiser* (June 7, 1969): xliv.

38. "Does 'The Pill' Still Need Estrogen?" Exluton trade literature, Organon (Thailand) Ltd, *c.* 1973, Syntex Files, Medical Science Collection, shows a 35-pill package; Micronor advertisement, *Journal of Obstetrics and Gynaecology of the British Commonwealth* (December 1972): iv, shows a 42-tablet "pushpak."

39. US Patent 5,020,671, "Method and Apparatus for Optimum Self-examination of Breasts by Users of Birth Control Pills," issued to Raleigh A. Smith, June 4, 1991.

40. Daron G. Ferris et al., "Effectiveness of Breast Self-examination Prompts on Oral Contraceptive Packaging," *The Journal of Family Practice* 42 (1996): 45.

41. US Patent 3,143,207, "Medication Dispensing Means," issued to David P. Wagner, August 4, 1964, col. 1, lines 52–56.

42. Leslie Aldridge Westoff and Charles F. Westoff, *From Now to Zero: Fertility, Contraception and Abortion in America* (Boston, 1971), pp. 109–10.

43. "Birth Control: The Pill and the Church," *Newsweek*, July 6, 1964.

44. Bakker and Dightman, "Psychological Factors in Fertility Control," *Fertility and Sterility* 15 (September/October 1964): 559–67, as reported in Edward E. Wallach and Celso-Ramón García, "Psychodynamic Aspects of Oral Contraception," *Journal of the American Medical Association* 203 (March 11, 1968): 927–30.

45. "Protect the New Patient from Her Own Forgetfulness," Lyndiol advertisement, Organon Laboratories Ltd of England, *Journal of Reproduction and Fertility* (November 1969): iv.

46. "Now You Can Give Her a 'Pill' that Really Counts for Her," Serial 28 advertisement, British Drug Houses (Canada) Ltd, *Canadian Medical Association Journal* 101 (November 29, 1969): 31.

47. Robert A. Hatcher et al., *Contraceptive Technology*, 16th rev. ed. (New York, 1994), p. 273; Juhn (n. 35 above), p. 33.

48. "Birth Control and the 11 P.M. News," *Philadelphia Daily News*, November 9, 1972.

49. Desogen, "Remember Me Compliance Kit," Medical Science Collections.

50. C. Wayne Bardin and Irving Sivin, "Norplant: The First Implantable Contraceptive," in *Contraception: Newer Pharmacological Agents, Devices, and Delivery Systems*, ed. Regine Sitruk-Ware and C. Wayne Bardin (New York, 1992), pp. 23–39; Brij B. Saxena and Mukul Singh, "Delivery of Contraceptive Drug by Subdermal Implants," in *Drug Delivery Devices: Fundamentals and Applications*, ed. Praveen Tyle (New York, 1988), pp. 302–21.

51. Helfand and Cowen, "Evolution of Pharmaceutical Oral Dosage Forms" (n. 19 above).

52. See Sheryl Burt Ruzek, *The Women's Health Movement: Feminist Alternatives to Medical Control* (New York, 1978); and The Boston Women's Health Book Collective, *Our Bodies, Ourselves* (New York, 1973).

53. John A. Robertson, *Children of Choice: Freedom and the New Reproductive Technologies* (Princeton, NJ, 1994), pp. 69–93, examines the social, ethical and legal consequences of Norplant.

54. Ellen Goodman, "The Politics of Norplant," *Washington Post*, February 19, 1991, p. A17.

55. Anita Hardon, "Norplant: Conflicting Views on its Safety and Acceptability," in *Issues in Reproductive Technology, An Anthology I*, ed. Helen Bequaert Holmes (New York, 1992), p. 27.

56. Tim Larimer, "Arming Girls Against Pregnancy," *USA Weekend*, February 26–28, 1993, p. 22.

57. Alexander Cockburn, "Norplant and the Social Cleansers, Part II," *The Nation*, July 25/ August 1, 1994, p. 116.

58. Anita Hardon (n. 55 above), pp. 11–30.

59. Dorothy L. Smith, "Compliance Packaging: A Patient Education Tool," *American Pharmacy* NS 29 (February 1989): 42–53.

60. Joel D. Howell's revealing account of the use of medical technologies in hospitals, *Technology in the Hospital: Transforming Patient Care in the Early Twentieth Century* (Baltimore, 1995), stresses the importance of the doctor–patient relationship in affecting the choice of technologies.

Timothy M. Boon

Histories, exhibitions, collections: Reflections on the language of medical curatorship at the Science Museum after Health Matters

The role of the curator in science museums is changing. As in previous decades of change, curators may resist, "go with the flow" or engage with the opportunities for change. Three interrelated questions encapsulate the current area of engagement: What styles of history should science museums employ in their accounts of the past? What styles of display should be adopted for the subjects we represent? What should we collect? By taking all three questions together it is possible to re-forge notions of curatorship in preparation for the decades to come. In this way we may preserve the best of what science museums have been as a foundation for what they may best become.

If, in the language of science museum curatorship, collections are the vocabulary, and history the grammar, then exhibition is the speech. Other curatorial cultures, such as those of the art museums, may have different "languages" because museum "languages," much like their literal counterparts, are historically determined. This essay is about the effect on our "speech" and "vocabulary" of adopting new "grammars." Or, to put it another way, we may change the exhibitions we create and the collections we hold if we recognise the range of historiographical possibilities open to us, and if we historicise our sense of exhibition. My argument here is not the assertion of a radical new possibility for curatorship, but the description of a process under way. I suggest that history, exhibition and collecting have, over the life of the Science Museum, London, always been intimately intertwined, but that, until recently, historiography has ranked low amongst curators' concerns. Here I shall look at issues surrounding the historiography of curatorial practice, before turning to historical aspects of exhibitions and collections. These sections form the basis for a discussion of approaches and methods applied in two recent medical exhibitions at the Science Museum, *Health Matters* and *Stories from the Germ Labs*. The arguments are mainly derived from experience of the Science Museum but they may also apply in a general sense to other similar institutions.

History in Science Museums: The Grammar of Curatorship
Specific historiographical views are necessarily contained in all museum work. This is not to say that previous generations of curators have always consciously espoused particular historiographies of science and technology, but rather that attitudes to the past are necessarily expressed in the

curatorial activities of exhibition and collecting. Many of these previous implicit historiographies were defined by exclusion, for example in the distinction drawn, since the Science Museum's first origins, between "historical" objects and "contemporary" ones, as recently explored by Xerxes Mazda.[1] In this view, the collections have always been, in large proportion, of obsolescent or superseded technologies. There is an important distinction, however, to be drawn between viewing objects as simply old, and seeing them as parts of potential historical narratives, and Mazda elucidates how the Museum, under different directors, took a more or less positive view of the historical accounts potentially present in the collections.[2]

We await a detailed study of the impact of past generations of curators on collections and exhibitions, but we may assume that they believed their worlds to have been transformed, in the classic industrial period, by technology and science. The evidence of the galleries and collections is that many of them continued to believe implicitly, and in an uncomplicated way, in the progress of science and technology.[3] Others outside museums, however, were voicing variants on the classical progressivist view in the inter-war period, and the products of curators may be contrasted with these. There is no outward sign, for example, of the inter-war radicalism associated with the "red professors," Bernal, Levy, Haldane and Hogben, being taken up and expressed in curatorial activities, even though the Science Museum hosted the 1931 conference which introduced the world to the Soviet delegation's Marxist interpretation of technological change.[4] Inter-war curators may also largely be distinguished from those activists troubled by the menace of modernisation, such as the smoke- and noise-abaters. Despite the fact that the Museum hosted two exhibitions originated by the voluntary health associations campaigning on these issues, and despite a curatorial presence on the organising committee of each, scarcely any history was visible within the exhibitions, which were mainly devoted to technical means of diagnosing and solving the problems. And, despite the fact that each boasted more than a hundred exhibits, no object already in the Museum's collections was used, and no new objects were subsequently acquired as a result of the exhibitions.[5]

Since the Second World War, the professional study of the history of science has changed beyond recognition. Globally, the histories of science, medicine and technology, with their various philosophical and policy siblings, have become established as mature, critical disciplines. To characterise them in brief invites caricature and omission,[6] but there has been a clear trend away from idealist, internalist accounts of sequences of scientific discoveries, which are the intellectual analogues of older styles of exhibition. Newer, more nuanced approaches have come to look at science as part of social life. First came the rejection of whiggism, defined as a tendency to write history as progress towards the present, rather than, as is now preferred, seeking to come to an understanding of how events were understood by contemporaries in the past. This rejection was followed by an analytical period concerned with scientific method and the nature of scientific change, exemplified by Thomas Kuhn's *The Structure of Scientific Revolutions*. In the 1970s, the social history of science, especially of its institutions, began to be widely discussed. At the same time, the implications of Foucault's radical synchronous view of history and his power-centred conception of knowledge began to make an impact, more in the history of medicine perhaps, than in the histories of science and technology.[7] The sociological analyses of science, particularly the "Edinburgh School" of social constructionism and the ethnomethodological wing, which has been expressed especially in studies of laboratory life, have provided the tools by which history of science has been able to pursue the social through to the construction of scientific facts themselves.[8] For science museum curators this potentially amounts to the invention of a series of new "grammars" with which they can "speak" in their core activities.

It would be naive, however, to suppose that changing curatorial practice is solely a matter of rational choice. Curators in science museums have experienced novel pressures in the last past decade, and the historiographies they espouse are changing in response to these, not simply because alternative historiographies exist, or because increasing numbers of curators are trained in historical disciplines. Some of these changes are associated with the changing priorities of institutions, which have produced redefinitions of curatorial responsibilities. The level of activity on the Royal Society's Public Understanding of Science initiative, for example, has resharpened the distinction between responsibilities to contemporary science and to its history, now read as a distinction between public understanding of science (think of the close analogue "health promotion") and contextual social history of science.

Another cultural pressure comes from the ubiquity of popular visual media, especially television, and the new interactive computer media. The various conventions of representing science and history on television and in the cinema may well affect the expectations of visitors to museums. Where our publics have both a visual literacy and knowledge drawn from these media, expectations of museums, and therefore of the curatorial role, are bound also to change.[9] Here again, a proper sense of the varieties of historical explanation may incline us to engage actively with some of the potential impacts of popular visual literacy. It is arguable that some broadcast genres are intellectual analogues of historiographical approaches: "fly on the wall" documentary may sit quite happily with ethnomethodology, for example, or "biopic" may be seen as a variant of biography no more distorting than many recent published examples. The question for curators relates to whether these modes should be translated into displays, and if not, what impact may be anticipated in public responses to our work? If it is right to produce more socially embedded accounts of our subjects than our predecessors did, then surely it is appropriate to reflect on the influence of visual media on our visitors' expectations. CD-ROM and World Wide Web media present us with similar challenges to make available our collections to new and larger audiences, but once again the interesting and unanswered questions relate to what types of account are appropriate, and what genres of interpretation should be used. Surely the means to gain fluency in this new form of "speech" is in the application of the historical "grammars" we already know and those we are willing to learn. The role of curators here, as in exhibitions, will increasingly be to set a wide diversity of examples of the power of artefacts to fertilise the understanding of the past and the present.

This confluence of broadening historiographical possibilities and larger social change is analogous with Cannadine's argument in his now classic essay "The Present and the Past in the English Industrial Revolution," which showed how generations of economic historians have interpreted the Industrial Revolution according to the economic conditions of their own day. He suggested that it may be inescapable that, as historians, we do this.[10] In a post-modern twist on this interpretation, it can be argued not only that this has happened, but that it behoves historians actively to reinterpret the past according to opportunities provided by modern conditions.[11] The lessons for science museum curators are clear: each generation of curator has a duty to adopt changed historiographical approaches as they make displays and collections; we can work only on the basis of what seems right and culturally significant to us in our own period. Equally, we cannot hide behind the modes of historical enquiry appropriate to foregoing generations.

These considerations also apply to the question of how curators should concern themselves with contemporary science in the collections and exhibitions they curate. It is important that both scientific change and novel technologies are seen as the products of historical processes, and that the potential range of historical accounts is considered in the collection and display of such items. This approach could be described as a "history of the present," as contrasted with the major alternative approach, public understanding of science, which often seems content to explain abstract scientific principles without reference to their constituting context. Nevertheless, as argued above, such exhibitions do tacitly convey particular historiographies, for example that science is to be understood as pure and unaffected by the context of its production.

Exhibition: The Speech of Curatorship
If it is widely acknowledged that the work of the historical community has a great deal to offer science museums, it is not often so readily considered that museum exhibitions are a fruitful context for undertaking and publishing historical research. Whereas historical work in science museums may be expressed in a variety of media – catalogues, television, lectures,

tours, for example – it has been in exhibitions that curatorial historical exposition has been at its most visible to the public, and I shall concentrate on its expression through that medium. Until fairly recently, items from Science Museum collections have most often been used to tell essentially whiggish stories of technical evolution and scientific progress. The hand- and machine-tools displays for example, dating from the 1930s, seemed to be able to trace every then-modern tool back to a flint, and the *Children's Gallery* effortlessly traced the history of lighting from the flaming brand to the electric lamp.[12] A more sophisticated example of the older exhibition style based on historical scholarship is visible in the Science Museum's chemistry galleries opened in the mid 1970s. In this display, an established history of chemistry is presented. Where the exhibits are no longer extant or are elsewhere, then replicas – for example of Stephen Hales' pneumatic apparatus – have been substituted.[13] Here, the wish to present *the* history of chemistry must have been the dominant concern, and artefacts, even key artefacts, are present as illustrations to quite substantial amounts of text. This is a model of display in which visitors are expected to read the exhibits much as they would read an illustrated book. In a museum which prides itself on its diversity, it is valuable to be able to compare exhibitions from different eras, but recent work in the history of science suggests alternative accounts and new emphases in the stories we tell about the history of chemistry. This bore fruit in the *Petroleum*, *Plastics* and *Industrial Chemistry* galleries which opted to present more socially embedded accounts.

Curators' exhibition practices are being changed by acquaintance with the historiographies of science, technology and medicine. Equally, an understanding of the historical processes responsible for the modes of display found in science museums should bear fruit in changed forms of historical science exhibitions. This is important so that we may ensure that "the public space for science" – Alan Morton's phrase – has a sophisticated historical dimension.[14] Ghislaine Lawrence has described the several styles which have been actively appropriated over a century by curators and latterly by museum designers. These include, from the 1920s, pictorialism, consciously drawing on the new trade of shop-window display and, from the 1930s, organisation of gallery spaces into single narratives with chapters, focused to transmit propositional knowledge to educational groups and adults alike, measured from the late 1950s by particular types of survey methodology.[15] The culmination of these trends, she asserts, is an impersonal style in which connotations of "authority, neutrality and value free facts – in short, of information – and also of palatability" dominate. As she comments, "For the curator … who wants to convey the social reality of practice and the socially made nature of theory – who wants to show that these areas are contested, interest related, subject to conventionalised representation in the media … this exhibition style is hopelessly, utterly inappropriate."[16] This engagement with the values conveyed by museum exhibition style found fruit in *Health Matters* in ways I describe below.

Modern historical concerns, for their own sakes and applied reflexively to the curator's business of exhibition, potentially have a very liberating effect on new displays, but, whilst exhibition provides unique opportunities as a medium for the exposition of rich historical stories, curators are not immune from the interests of the other individuals and organisations involved. The argument of this paper relates rather to those aspects of the process which are within the curator's power to influence – that is, their creative representational decisions, so often the domain of unnecessary self-censorship.[17] Practical demands of exhibition space and suppositions about the behaviour of visitors may also affect what types of historical account may be employed. As this may be *terra incognita* for some readers, a limited comparison may help: the substrate of exhibition may be said to be three-dimensional space, where in literary productions it is two-dimensional space and in film it is time. Unlike cinema films or television programmes (but like video recordings and Web pages), museum exhibitions permit different sequences, speeds and levels of detail in viewing. Equally, they differ in being unable to command the narrative drive constructed by the directors and editors of conventional cinema narratives.[18] In common with films, books and video recordings, museum exhibitions have the potential to permit analytical and critical consumption, although in practice they seem rarely to be used in this way. This, no doubt, is a product of their different social and cultural location, in which traditions of exegesis and commentary have become attached to the published and written word and, to a lesser extent, to the moving image, as parts of scholarly activity – modes which currently have no commonly found equivalents for exhibitions, especially those concerned with "scientific" subjects.[19]

Collections: The Vocabulary of Curatorship

As with exhibitions, understanding that traditions of collecting are historically made may help us come to a better conception of how a sense of historiography may focus collections. When all that the museum owned was displayed, then we could say that collection and exhibition were the same thing. Since then, with the proliferation of off-site storage, collections have come to be considered as different in kind from exhibitions. But we do continue to define reserve collections in relation to exhibition – the "great undisplayed," if you like – but the arguments for reserve collections are linked to trends in display in a negative sense, too: the justification for reserve collections would diminish enormously, perhaps to vanishing point, if we were to remove museum objects from their central role in display and make them mere adjuncts to interactive exhibits. That is why vigorous arguments, not just about the importance of historical approaches to exhibition, but also about their potential breadth, impinge on our notions of collections.

As curators and designers alter their notions of exhibition design and narrative, reserve collections may tend to become stagnant backwaters, conforming to archaic notions, to last decade's collecting policy. Previous generations of curators did not always openly espouse a sophisticated historical approach in collecting policies, but, once again, a particular style of historical account – concerned with technical improvement, perhaps – may be implicit in the collections they amassed. There is a great temptation either to follow atavistically another generation's collecting practices, or else to make too much sense of what our forebears have left us – wishing to fill gaps in perceived sequences, or desiring to extend imagined series. As time passes, curators may gain the impression that the reserve collection represents some absolute set which, obeying some natural order, is able to sit separate from exhibition as a superordinate, pure entity.

At its most extreme, this may be seen in the typological collections of technical museums which seem to imply, for example, that if we have every type of X-ray tube, both gas and Coolidge, stationary anode and rotating, air-, water- or gas-cooled, diagnostic as well as therapeutic, then we shall be able to tell the history of X-rays.[20] Well actually, no. For *Health Matters,* in addition to an X-ray machine, we needed a fire extinguisher, a doctor's coat, stethoscope and textbook, some trade literature in an old suitcase, and a bowl of mashed potato. The reason for this is that history of medicine and history of technology, as they have incorporated more social history over the past 40 years, have made it both necessary and possible to create a much more nuanced account of technical change. Here was a standard ward X-ray set making the argument that radiology was the only widespread electrical medical technology in the inter-war period, abetted by the fire extinguisher, a signifier for the messy social history of X-ray practice, in which nitrate films caused several major fires in X-ray departments. The doctor's effects signify the argument between medical believers in the clinical art and champions of the new machine diagnosis. The trade literature in a suitcase represents the machine as a commodity bought by hospitals and sold by companies. The mashed potato, which acted as a vehicle for early contrast media for radiographs of the gut is an indicator of the patient's experience.

The argument suggested by this example is that changing modes of historical understanding are altering what we consider to be significant. As we must collect what we view as significant, we shall renew our collections by the addition of new categories of object in response to the intense engagement with representational issues which arises when producing exhibitions. This way of thinking about acquisition can lead to uncomfortable conclusions, especially over the differential inventory status of objects;[21] for example, by definition we cannot have real mashed potato from the pre-war period, and the value traditionally placed on authenticity forbids us from assigning to the replica the status of an inventoried object. This is not a trivial point as we seek to represent from the past aspects of material culture not considered important by our predecessors. A partial solution lies in redirecting our discomfort to reflect on how else we might represent these aspects of the history of X-rays: are there remnants of the literature used to inform patients about contrast media, for example, or what do patients' diaries record of the experience? By reflecting on these types of issues, we may actively feed back into our collecting policies new perceptions generated by the intensive historical work of exhibition production, so that we may acquire categories of object which can be collected only slowly over time.

We can, however, go beyond these practical day-to-day concerns to retune our understanding of what a collection is. There are distinct benefits to be accrued from returning to seeing collections as forms of representation similar to exhibitions. We may imagine the worlds that the collection as it stands potentially represents, and consider the impact on that representation of adding new categories of object. We have been moving away from exhibitions as displays of existent collections, partially because the collections we curate have been unable to supply the objects that we need to tell particular types of stories in displays – the absence of a good collection of twentieth-century vaccines acted as a brake on the historical account in *Health Matters*, for example. The circumstances of the headlong rush of gallery creation are far from ideal for extending the breadth of collections, but there is a need to apply the exhibition style of thought to the improvement of collections in periods of "normal curatorship", to adopt a Kuhnian metaphor. This is not to suggest that we are able to anticipate what may be needed for displays in the future. Rather, it suggests that applying our knowledge of what has proved useful in the present may be used as a model for the types of items we should lay up as resources for the future.

The Wellcome Collections provide a telling lesson of how different the assumptions underlying collecting have been in the past. They were accumulated mainly in fulfilment of an evidential purpose, obsolescent even at the time, to provide the basis for a materialist anthropologico-historical account of human development.[22] Within this project, not only did Henry Wellcome collect categories of objects outside conventional notions of medicine and healing, but he was content with copies and replicas. Only very late in the day, with the "French Collection", did he collect according to the biographical mode – acquiring the effects of scientists and doctors – one of the governing preoccupations of modernistic curatorship.[23] Here again, the categories were broad: Curie certainly, but also dozens of now generally forgotten minor physicians and chemists.[24] This contrasts with the range of collecting styles now extant in medical, scientific and technological collections: anthropological, biographical, serial/technical, social-historical (as in Trevelyan – collecting the remains of previous social life), "mythological" (in the sense that an artefact can be collected with the intention of using it in display as the crux of a dichotomy[25]); social constructivist (on the basis that reality is made in social relations) and, quite possibly, others. But, just because items were collected for different reasons than we might now choose, it does not follow that the resulting collections are irrelevant to our current purposes. We daily put new complexions on the potential meanings of the collections. To give just one example, the 10,000 non-Western artefacts held in the Wellcome collections at this museum may now, reflexively, be seen as evidence of the endeavour to come to terms with non-Western peoples in an age of empire. This raises the possibility of collecting more material associated with the practice of anthropology, a science outside the established interests of the Science Museum. As a result of considerations of this nature, a small start has been made in improving our holdings of anthropometrical instruments.

Health Matters

Health Matters, the Science Museum's gallery devoted to twentieth-century medicine, offered both an opportunity to apply some of the critical notions developed in preceding years, and a site for their further development. This section of the paper gives a description of the gallery and highlights examples of how the styles of thought described above affected choices during the production of the gallery. As I proceed, I shall discuss the ways in which it can be seen as an expression of recent historiographical debates, and the light it sheds on the opportunities and difficulties thrown up by our approach. Briefly, of the categories discussed above, medical collecting inspired by the social-historical principles of modern history of science had been developing for a decade before the gallery received approval for production to begin, in late 1991. On the other hand, in terms of display, the Museum had been through a period of directing its resources away from temporary exhibitions, but a great deal of theoretical and historical work on exhibitions had been undertaken, both in internal discussions about new medical galleries planned but not executed, and in the published work of senior project curator, Ghislaine Lawrence.[26] *Health Matters* was the culmination of this work; it was envisaged as a departure from typological exhibitions (such as the Museum's *Optics* display), as eschewing narratives of technical development (present in the former *Land Transport* galleries) and as having an approach different from the didacticism championed by the exhibit development team of the Natural History Museum (and expressed in the Science Museum's *Food for Thought* gallery). It was designed to engage with and represent the social realities of clinical medicine, public health and medical science, and to follow the spirit of recent debates by favouring narratives other than those of technical development. It therefore gave priority to the representation of themes often absent from medical displays: the nature of scientific work, the patient's experience of medicine, and medicine as reported and understood through the lens of popular media, for example. By means of appropriately vivid and involving media of communication it was intended to convey to the visitor a rich and compelling story of the recent history of medicine as it has been experienced in the past half century.

Opened in June 1994, the gallery was the product of a two-and-a-half year, full-time project, which itself followed more than five years of part-time proposal writing and sponsorship chasing. It was always a curatorial project, but in its implementation a multidisciplinary team of about 20 – curators, researchers, designers, audio-visual producers, project managers and building contractors – was employed.[27] Corporately, the Museum had decided to produce a gallery on modern medicine for two reasons: historical coverage and display style. First, we wanted to complement the two Wellcome galleries of the history of medicine, *The Science and Art of Medicine* (1981) which uses about 3,000 museum objects and text panels to convey a substantial history and anthropology of medicine in objects "from Plato to NATO," and *Glimpses of Medical History* (1980) which uses the display technologies of the diorama and the room set to introduce the subject. Within their long historical coverage, neither of these galleries is able to discuss modern medicine in great depth. In addition, the former gallery is very much in the "history of ideas" tradition; its conventional object density, text length and subdued lighting convey a sense of sobriety, almost of awe, in the presence of the long history of medicine.

Historiographical focus and exhibition style are not independent variables, however. Because museum visitors carry with them knowledge and expectations of the appearance of science exhibitions, it is appropriate for exhibitions presenting facets of subjects not normally represented in this medium to do so by means of different display techniques. *Health Matters* engages with established notions of medical and scientific museum display on a broad front. It was an unspoken ethos of the project that no display convention would be used without question. This is illustrated in this paragraph from the design brief:

It might be helpful to make some general points here about what we do *not* want: The style should avoid being didactic, neutral, or of a type often associated with health education or human biology.[28] The gallery will not be heavily reliant on objects in cases and we would hope to avoid spaces highly divided by vertical screens/panels. We hope that text will not automatically be placed in blocks on panels; it might be elsewhere – on objects, even? Technical information of the "how it works type" will not normally be incorporated in the display, but will be made available on leaflets in the gallery. Static and moving images should be large and atmospheric with minimal use of small monitors. If it were an art display, it might be closer to an "installation" than to a "hanging."

In conclusion, we suggested some of the words which we would be happy to see associated with this gallery, and the socio-historical account of modern medicine it would display:

documentary; ambience; impressions; ethnography; personal experience; humour; spectacle; surprise; juxtapositions; questions.[29]

This demonstrates at the least a determination to see the problem of display and that of style of historical account as intimately entwined. Nevertheless, to make such a statement is to underplay the heuristic of producing the gallery, the adventure which clarified many of these issues.

Section One of *Health Matters – The rise of medicine –* concentrates on the machines and medicines which now characterise the clinical encounter between the individual patient and the medical doctor, the individual representative of modern medicine. One of the crossovers between historiography and display technique was in the choice of stories, some of which focused on aspects of recent medicine which were expected to be surprising to the visitor: you may see here, for example, the connection between the Mexican yam and contraceptives, or sausages and kidney machines. This is not mere flippancy, but a means of representing the highly contingent and socially embedded nature of the development of modern medicine. One post-war cardiac surgery technique, for example, borrowed process-engineering techniques from ice-cream manufacture.[30] Juxtaposition became one of our main techniques here – of familiar with unfamiliar, or of things which would not immediately seem to belong in the same category. By these means, for those who wished to engage with a further level of detail, multiple historical narratives could be "spun off" the core exhibits of the gallery. An example is the display of an iron lung with the wheel from a 1935 Morris Eight car as a means of providing a "hook" for a story about what types of organisations produced medical machines in the inter-war period, and more distantly, about the absence at that time of any highly developed medical technology industry (with the exception of manufacturers of X-ray and electro-medical equipment).

Another crossover of this type arose in the way in which the archive films in this section were selected. Historical awareness of the mode of address of different genres of film, and a critical response to the ways in which film is often used naively in museum displays, led to a close engagement with the potential of the material viewed during research.[31] Just as the objects shown were to be authentic, so the visitors were to see authentic contemporary film footage, not the highly reconfigured "wallpaper" of much current television documentary. This was felt to be important because the re-editing of archive material is liable to obliterate its "mode of address," which conveys much of the meaning understood by audiences.[32] But here, two remote aspects of the gallery's approach collided. The strategy of the gallery was, by enlarging the communicative media to include the non-verbal aspects of architecture and design, to reduce reliance on the printed, displayed word; accordingly, display panels were limited to 60 words, rather than the more usual 100 words or more. Similarly, and for practical reasons, sequences of film were limited to 90 seconds per object.[33] Of all the hundred or more films of a dozen types viewed for the gallery, one genre in particular lent itself to display in gallery circumstances, namely Newsreel. This genre, marked by its characteristics of constant commentary, light orchestral music and upbeat accounts of virtually all subjects, had originally been designed primarily to be shown to people who did not wish to see it – the audiences for feature films, to whom it was shown as part of larger programmes.[34] For *Health Matters*, it fulfilled a requirement to illustrate reportage, and to display the conventions under which medical technology has been represented, with all the rich verbal and non-verbal cargo the medium conveys. Both the fact that it was originally designed to appeal to the general public, and the consequential rapid editing, made it more satisfactory when cut still further, for gallery purposes, than slower-paced, less facetious genres – documentary, for example. Even in this already highly compressed material, we were obliged to make significant cuts: the 1964 Pathé story, "Artificial kidney saves wife's life," was cut to one-third of its original length. For our purposes here, the significance of this process is the manner in which it affected the range of historical accounts presented in the gallery. Where documentaries might have told socially attuned stories of social conditions, features might have told heroic stories of individuals' triumph over suffering, and technical films aimed at doctors might have shown doctors how to undertake particular procedures.[35] Newsreel coverage of medical technology tended to be focused on clever scientists, technical marvels, plucky patients and, occasionally, eccentric inventors. Where such material is favoured for practical reasons, as has happened in some cases in *Health Matters*, it may often not be read by visitors as an ironic, historically contingent style, but as a reinforcement of received views of scientific and technical change.[36]

Section Two – *The rise of health* – is concerned with the ways in which the study of the health of populations – rather than individuals – has transformed our ideas of health in half a century. Here, the impact of historiographical concerns may be seen more in the types of subjects chosen for treatment and the emphasis given to them than in any popularisation of existing work. Compared with the amount published on the histories of clinical and laboratory medicine, twentieth-century, and especially post-war, public health lacks a substantial mature historical literature, although this is beginning to be rectified. This may explain why the selection of historical exhibits owes more than we realised at the time to David Armstrong's Foucauldian account of social medicine.[37] But the concerns of these displays – with the history of public health as the history of surveillance, with the historically contingent nature of the idea of positive health, with the relationships between scientific and lay groups, and with epidemiology as a type of work – are all typical of mainstream modern history of medicine and science. As in the remainder of the gallery, *The rise of health* uses examples to convey dominant themes of twentieth-century medicine. There are three historical displays – on Arnold Gesell's work establishing norms of child development, on the Peckham Health Centre as site of surveillance of health, and on the establishment of a link between smoking and lung cancer – and a separate cone-shaped area containing artist-designed interactive exhibits on the nature and content of contemporary epidemiology. More than in other gallery sections, the degree of abstraction of the subject matter forced us to develop new means of representing important historical themes where, had we relied on the collection as it stood, we should have been unable to mount a display at all. For example, the display on the epidemiology of smoking uses the juxtaposition of a seductive 1950s cigarette advertisement and the brute technology of epidemiological work: the punched-card sorter and the calculating machine.[38] This is a concrete example of how the creative representational work of exhibition production may help to redirect collecting policies: the technology of epidemiology continues to be a collecting concern.

Section Three – *Science in medicine* – portrays the way in which we now turn to science for the answers to medical problems, in a way that took the best part of a century to establish: our understanding of disease processes is now founded in molecular genetics, in DNA.[39] *Health Matters* invites the visitor to reflect on this fact, but it also draws on the work of Latour and Woolgar to encourage reflection on the nature of medical laboratory work.[40] An introductory space juxtaposes Crick and Watson's 1953 molecular model of DNA with molecular motifs in 1950s society – such as designs from the Festival of Britain – and modern uses of DNA iconography. One conceptual thread then introduces the idea of the use of cells and micro-organisms as tools of medical laboratory work, both in exhibits, and in a wall-filling mural by Borin van Loon, whose work may be familiar to readers from the *Beginner's Guide* series of books. Another thread picks up the promise to take an ethnographic view of our subjects by representing laboratory work, in a group of exhibits which includes: four artists' exact replications of scientists' desks, produced by Matthew Dalziel and Louise Scullion (*see* Figure 1); large reproductions of laboratory daybooks; machines used to visualise molecules; and a spoof radio interview by Tony Hawks deconstructing the language of scientific publication. Linking this section to the end is "the street," part hyperreal representation of a street, part referential reportage photomontage, designed to be a reminder of the "real world" in which people have diseases, and in which medical research is undertaken. The gallery is completed by a sound–slide–object programme which looks at AIDS, cancer and heart disease, using a variety of lay and medical viewpoints. Where older style exhibits might have concentrated on technical details of aetiology or mode of infection, this approach is "in the round" of social reality, implying that what each of these diseases may be is dependent on the viewpoint adopted. This display acts as a composite summary of the viewpoints of the gallery's three sections.

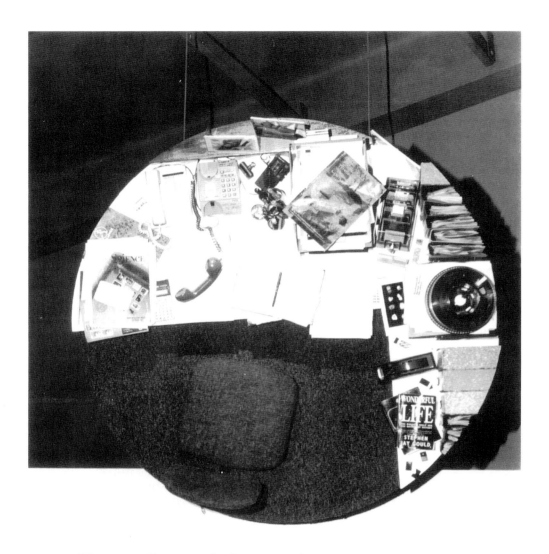

Chester Beatty Laboratories,
Institute of Cancer Research,
London, 4.30 pm
15th November 1993

Figure 1. Laboratory sculpture by Dalziel and Scullion from Section Three of the Health Matters *gallery,* Science in medicine.

Stories from the Germ Labs

Health Matters was built with a final room which has become the location for a series of temporary exhibitions on subjects related to the themes of the main display, starting with an exhibition of specially commissioned photographs by Clive Boursnell. There have followed *Bedpan Art* which, picking up the use of artists' work in the larger display, showed artworks produced by students using manufacturers' reject disposable bedpans; *50 Years of Penicillin*, which was the expression in exhibition form of some of Robert Bud's recent work on the historical iconography of penicillin;[41] and *Thicker than Water*, which, drawing on Kim Pelis' historical research project, looked at the ambiguous nature of blood in an exhibition to mark the 50th anniversary of the National Blood Transfusion Service. The largest of these "updates," situated in a new temporary exhibition area in the Lower Wellcome Gallery, is *Stories from the Germ Labs*, which marks 50 years of the Public Health Laboratory Service (PHLS).[42] Here was a subject which was congruent with our long-term aim to improve the representation of modern public health activity in exhibitions and collections, which was also potentially of great public interest: a state-financed organisation, scarcely known by name to the majority of the population, which touches the life of every individual, not only through responses to epidemics, but also through direct intervention in the lives of millions, for example in the childhood immunisation programmes which the PHLS administers. The exhibition takes a cool and gently humorous look at our cohabitation with infectious organisms over the past half century, a period which stretches from the pre-antibiotic era to what some may consider the post-antibiotic age.

Of all historical genres, specific institutional history is perhaps the least suited to a public exhibition. So, when we were approached by the PHLS, it was clear that, if it were to be a successful public display, important decisions had to be made about its style and about the organisation of material within it. Here, an explicitly historiographical choice was being made. The first decision was to structure the exhibition material using a journalistic metaphor of stories, as the polar opposite of a chronological account of institutional development. Each "story" was required to have a degree of cultural resonance or humour to catch the attention of the visitor. The aim was to present multiple narratives, each different in kind, and each touching on an aspect of the history of the PHLS, from its Second World War foundation as the *Emergency* PHLS to some recent threatened or real epidemics. Contained in this multiplicity of narratives is a metaphor for the diversity of possible historical accounts of the subject.[43]

In addition to the name given to the exhibition, several techniques were used to convey the idea of narratives. Display panels in *Stories from the Germ Labs* adopt the iconography of a tabloid newspaper, using a red masthead version of the title, and typically flippant headlines. Taking the opposite approach to text length from that in *Health Matters*, and intending to capitalise on the metaphor of the journalistic story, these newspaper "stories" sometimes exceed 300 words. Here the implication is not that the visitor might be expected to read everything in the exhibition, but rather that they are expected to skip through and just read what takes their fancy. The atmosphere of narrative is heightened by the four film clips, three of which use music which implies narrative: *Sugar Lump Vaccine*, on the 1961 Hull polio vaccination campaign, has the light orchestral score of a newsreel; *Surprise Attack*, advocating smallpox vaccination, has a Rachmaninov-style tone; and *Another Case of Poisoning*, on food poisoning, has a spiky atonal score. This density of the panels is also found in the displays themselves which, as in *Health Matters*, use small objects to signify larger stories – toy trains and planes signifying social change, transport of people and of diseases, for example.

In addition to the eight "stories" given their own displays, there are several themes which recur throughout the exhibition. One is hygiene, the making of boundaries between the clean and the unclean, and of hand washing; the culture, as Mary Douglas would say, of "matter out of place."[44] Accordingly, surrealism, the art form most closely associated with juxtaposition for effect, and therefore of "matter out of place" seemed the ideal display style. As a result, it is not bacteria or viruses that are shown in the "Porton" microbiological manipulation cabinet, but examples of popular books, novels and videotapes about "killer bugs" (*see* Figure 2). In the display on MRSA (Methicillin Resistant Staphyloccus Aureus, currently a substantial cause of hospital infections), a pair of disembodied hands reaches out of a model hospital to wash itself in a passing basin. Here, we feel, is a sense of "appropriate" display style which is different in conception from the "neutrality" of many science displays.[45] It also raises the question of the wider range of responses which a science exhibition might hope to provoke, beyond studiousness or cheerful assimilation of facts. The signifier group used to introduce the topic of PHLS checks for polio contamination in sea water includes, amongst sand and saucy postcards, something which might be a piece of human excrement, wearing sunglasses, in a seaside bucket. Here is a dense connotative display which alludes to well-established traditions of specifically British humour, relocating science where it belongs in a dense web of lived social experience, rather than abstracting a pure scientific conclusion, an organism count. Before a word is read, it signifies the import of one small part of the work of the PHLS, namely their studies of the microbiological safety of bathing waters. It may also, for some visitors, provoke a guffaw. Humour, beyond a very limited range, has not been much used in science displays,[46] and one must conclude that it has been deemed inappropriate for a "serious" subject; or it may be that its anarchic tendencies not to appeal to all museum visitors equally makes it unsuitable as if, because they fit the same socio-economic categories, visitors might be considered to have identical experience of life. Have we, in an attempt not to offend those who may not "get" every joke,

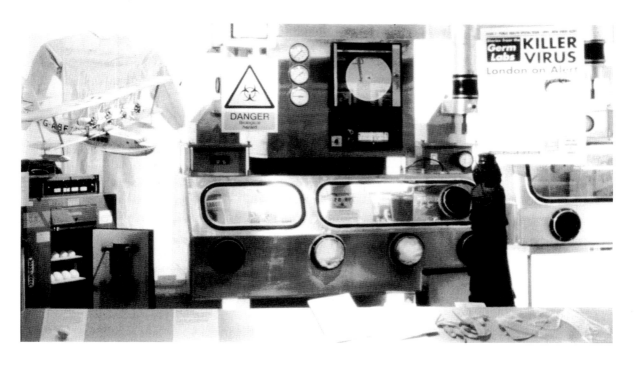

Figure 2. "Killer Virus: London on Alert," One of the Stories from the Germ Labs.

deprived ourselves of a powerful tool in museum display? It must be the case that the ways in which the lay public expect to "read" science displays are deeply ingrained because of the conventions of science-popularising discourse in other media. This is not a reason to refrain from breaking out from those conventions; indeed, such breaking out may be necessary if the real scientific literacy of the population is to improve.

The exhibition's other main underlying theme is the world view of infectious-disease epidemiologists. Like historians who have taken the Darwinian turn, these scientists are concerned with social change large and small, not for its own sake, but because of the opportunities it provides for differential bacterial growth and viral spread. This is evident, for example, in a story under the heading "An Outbreak of Semolina Poisoning." This retells the story of the PHLS's investigation of an episode of food poisoning spread by bacterial growth in chocolate semolina pudding which had been centrally produced and distributed to Devon schools in 1947.[47] The display incorporates a speech by G. S. Wilson, Director of the PHLS, on how the growth of mass catering was providing new opportunities for the spread of bacterial diseases.[48] As in the third section of *Health Matters*, it was felt that one important task of an exhibition of contemporary history is to convey some general characteristics, almost in an anthropological sense, of working scientists, doing what a Kuhnian would describe as "normal science." The associations of the bacteriological investigation of school dinners, mingling slight disgust with gentle humour, make an ideal "hook" for this theme, which is picked up in the portfolio of photographs commissioned from photojournalist David Modell. This follows a potentially infected food sample in its journey from factory to PHLS headquarters. These photographs are now part of the permanent collection, and represent a collecting initiative in representing the process of science within public health.

Conclusion

Historiography, collecting and exhibition are mutually dependant activities. If a sociologist's or a historian's concern with "laboratory life" means that we can think about how we seek to represent the practice of science, then we must take the opportunity both in display and in collecting. So, for example, the opportunity was taken with *Stories from the Germ Labs* to collect and show a "Porton" cabinet for sterile manipulation of dangerous micro-organisms. If public exhibition requires that we investigate medical technology (say) from a new standpoint – the "biography" of a kidney machine and its owner, or the commercial policies of first-generation medical technology manufacturers – then we should introduce some of these concerns into the historical mainstream.[49] If the practicalities of historical display require us to display items we do not hold in our collections, then we must, reflexively, modify our collecting policies so that there is a smaller chance of future displays being dominated by obsolescent collecting practices. Alternatively, the historical contingencies of past collecting may themselves have something to say about the relative social location of museums and medicine which would be worth discussing both in displays and in scholarly work; the breadth of the original Wellcome collections might be a good example here. Collections, historiography and exhibition together make up curatorship as vocabulary, grammar and speech are constitutive of language. Each element may alter another and each must be permitted to change under another's influence.

Notes

1. X. Mazda, "The Changing Role of History in the Policy and Collections of the Science Museum, 1857–1973," Unpublished ms., *Science Museum Papers in the History of Technology* no. 3 (London, 1996). For a deconstruction of notions of contemporaneity, see S. Schaffer, "Temporary Contemporary: Some Puzzles of Science in Action," in *Here and Now: Contemporary Science and Technology in Museums and Science Centres,* ed. G. Farmelo and J. Carding (London, 1997), pp. 31–39.
2. This is not intended to deny that some of the Museum's founding collections were acquired because they were considered to be of historical importance. Bennet Woodcroft's Patent Office Collection contained items such as Stephenson's *Rocket*, already a feature of Smilesian narratives of technological change. See the introduction to N. Cossons, A. Nahum, and P. Turvey, eds, *Making of the Modern World: Milestones of Science and Technology* (London, 1992).
3. A nuanced account of the origins of Science Museum representations of physics is given in: A. Morton, "The Electron Made Public: Pure Science at the British Empire Exhibition, 1924–25", *Artefacts* 2 (forthcoming).
4. See G. Werskey, ed., *Science at the Cross Roads: Papers Presented to the International Congress of the History of Science and Technology, held in London from June 29th to July 3rd, 1931, by Delegates of the U.S.S.R.,* 2nd ed. (London, 1971); G. Werskey, *The Visible College,* 2nd ed. (London, 1988).

5. These conclusions are drawn on the evidence of the catalogues: Anti-Noise League, *Noise Abatement Exhibition* (London, 1935); National Smoke Abatement Society, *Smoke Abatement Exhibition Handbook and Guide* (Manchester, 1936) and Science Museum nominal files 5134 (Noise abatement) and 5397A (Smoke abatement). For the context of the 1930s smoke debate see T. M. Boon, "The Smoke Menace: Cinema, Sponsorship, and the Social Relations of Science in 1937," in *Science and Nature (British Society for the History of Science Monograph 8)*, ed. M. Shortland (Oxford, 1993), pp. 57–88.

6. For a more detailed view, see the first section of R. Olby, G. Cantor, J. Christie, and M. Hodge, eds., *Companion to the History of Modern Science* (London, 1990). J. Christie, "The Development of the Historiography of Science," pp. 5–22, gives a sophisticated account of the longer historiography of science.

7. See C. Jones and R. Porter, eds., *Reassessing Foucault: Power, Medicine and the Body* (London, 1994).

8. In general see T. Pinch, "The Sociology of the Scientific Community," in R. Olby et al., eds. (n. 6 above), pp. 87–99. For a specific example, see B. Latour, *Science in Action* (Milton Keynes, 1987).

9. A case study of the implications of differences between television and museum as media is to be found in G. Lawrence, "Object Lessons in the Museum Medium", *New Research in Museum Studies: Objects of Knowledge* 1 (1990): 103–24.

10. D. Cannadine, "The Present and the Past in the English Industrial Revolution," *Past and Present* 103 (1984): 131–72.

11. This twist was suggested to me by Prof. Ulrich Wengenroth.

12. Each maquette was, confusingly, illuminated by an electrical light bulb.

13. Either those made for this exhibition, or for previous displays based on similar assumptions. This display may still be seen on the second floor of the Museum.

14. Morton gives examples of the Special Loan Exhibition of 1876 and the British Empire Exhibition of 1924. A. Morton, "Curatorial Challenges: Contexts, Controversies and Things," in G. Farmelo and J. Carding, eds. (n. 1 above), pp. 147–54, but similar arguments also apply instructively to, say, the 1951 Festival of Britain, for which, see S. Forgan, "Festivals of Science and the Two Cultures: Science, Design and Display in the Festival of Britain 1951," *British Journal for the History of Science*, 31 (1998): 217–40.

15. On evaluation, see G. Lawrence, "Rats, Street Gangs and Culture: Evaluation in Museums," in *Museum Languages: Objects and Texts*, ed. G. Kavanagh (Leicester, 1991), pp. 11–32.

16. G. Lawrence, "Museums and the Spectacular," in *Museums and Late Twentieth Century Culture: Transcripts taken from a Series of Lectures given at the University of Manchester, October–December 1994* (Manchester, 1994), pp. 69–82, 75.

17. Self censorship by the Food Gallery project team was one of the themes noted by Sharon Macdonald; S. MacDonald and R. Silverstone, "Science on Display: The Representation of Scientific Controversy in Museums," *Public Understanding of Science* 1 (1992): 69–87.

18. This is so even when a cinematic model seems to be at work, for example in the *Wooden Walls* exhibition at Chatham Historic Dockyard, which employs a series of electrical, electronic and mechanical techniques to tell the story of one apprentice's experience in the ship-building yard during the construction of one particular warship. Also, there are influential traditions of experimental film-making which seek to disrupt the traditional techniques of cinematic narrative; see, for example, the work of Chris Marker, and of the French *Nouvelle Vague*.

19. Although there has recently been a great increase in analytical museological publication (see for example the *New Research in Museum Studies* series), this has yet to make much of a dent in newspaper and magazine responses to museum displays, where science exhibitions in particular suffer from falling between the responsibilities of art, design, science and health journalists.

20. There may, of course, be other uses which would justify such acquisitions; my argument is about what else we should collect.

21. There is a continuing ontological debate about what categories of object should be considered appropriate to become inventoried museum objects. Here, at some stages in our history, we have operated a type of "apartheid": "significant" objects may gain the status of being on the Museum's official inventory, with the legal status that goes with it. This is the theory of inventory status as membership of "the Elect". How much more fruitful might it be

to give the same status to all objects which can support narratives of change within science. This is a model in which we collect more in anticipation of building new understandings in future, or in anticipation of later weeding and disposal.

22. G. Skinner, "Sir Henry Wellcome's Museum for the Science of History," *Medical History* 30 (1986): 383–418.

23. L. Ward, "The Cult of Relics: Pasteur Material at the Science Museum," *Medical History* 38 (1994): 52–72.

24. *French Material*, typescript catalogue in archives of Wellcome Institute, copy held at Science Museum.

25. R. Bud, "Science, Meaning and Myth in the Museum", *Public Understanding of Science* 4 (1995): 1–16.

26. See notes 9, 15, 16 and 22.

27. Led by Ghislaine Lawrence, with the assistance of the current author, designed by Jasper Jacob, with audio-visual production by Triangle Two. The principal sponsor was SmithKline Beecham, and patrons were Action Research, British Diabetic Association, British Heart Foundation, Medical Research Council, The Multiple Sclerosis Society and the Wellcome Trust.

28. It was argued that to adopt the design style of health education would be to assume the identity of a subject which, within the historical approach of the gallery, should be a subject for analysis.

29. One member of the design team later confessed that this was one of the most difficult briefs they had ever received.

30. Ghislaine Lawrence, "Design Solutions for Medical Technology: Charles Drew's Profound Hypothermia Apparatus for Cardiac Surgery," this volume, pp. 63–77.

31. This is too complex a subject to cover in this paper but, to take one example, commercial films or videotapes designed to sell commodities are often used in museum displays without reflection on the impression conveyed to the visitor.

32. This arose from the current author's historical work on health films; see for example: T. Boon, "Citizenship, Public Health and Mode of Address: The Public Health Campaigns of the Ministry of Health, 1939–45," unpublished paper given to "The Right to Health in Modern Society" conference, Oxford, July 11–12, 1997. See also reference quoted in note 5 above.

33. Of the eight projectors running as four pairs in Section One, two at a time show 90 seconds of full motion video followed by four-and-a-half minutes of repeated sequences of silent stills. Thus any visitor has to wait six minutes for any one sequence to "come round" again. (This was the compromise reached to reduce problems of "crosstalk" between displays).

34. See, for an example of historical literature on this genre, T. Aldgate, "The Newsreels, Public Order and the Projection of Britain," in *Impacts and Influences: Essays on Media Power in the Twentieth Century*, ed. J. Curran, A. Smith, and P. Wingate (London, 1987), pp. 145–56.

35. As the Allen & Hanburys financed *Profound Hypothermia* film did for hypothermic heart surgery.

36. Visitors' comment books from *Health Matters* revealed that visitors' positivist assumptions about science and technology led them to read the gallery as a confirmation of pre-existing views. This should be of no surprise to historians, but it does beg questions of just how challenging displays would have to become before they impinged directly on visitors' expectations.

37. D. Armstrong, *Political Anatomy of the Body* (Cambridge, 1983).

38. Here, the execution falls short of the conception, both in the size of the poster reproduction, and in the omission of a neon sign, intended to bring in a whole raft of extra connotations, for which see Lawrence (n. 16 above), p. 76.

39. For a good introduction for this transformation, see A. Cunningham and P. Williams, eds., *The Laboratory Revolution in Medicine* (Cambridge, 1992).

40. Latour, B., *Science in Action: How to Follow Scientists and Engineers through Society* (Milton Keynes, 1987); B. Latour and S. Woolgar, *Laboratory Life: The Social Construction of Scientific Facts*, (London, 1979).

41. R. Bud, "Penicillin and the New Elizabethans", *British Journal for the History of Science* (forthcoming, 1998).

42. The exhibition was produced in collaboration with the PHLS, via their head of Press and PR (but with editorial control in the Museum's hands) and sponsored by NatWest Corporate Banking Services. It was curated by the current author, designed by Peter Davison of the Museum's Design Office, with research by Sarah Angliss.

43. Narratives were selected from the organisation's official history [R. Williams, *Microbiology for the Public Health: The Evolution of the Public Health Laboratory Service, 1939–1980* (London, 1985)] and from suggestions made by PHLS staff.

44. M. Douglas, *Purity and Danger* (London, 1966).

45. Both Lawrence (n. 16 above), p. 78, and Schaffer (n. 1 above), p. 38, also comment on juxtaposition and surrealism.

46. Lawrence (n. 16 above), p. 78.

47. The scientific report is: B. Moore, "A Food-poisoning Outbreak Apparently Caused by α-Haemolytic Streptococci," *Monthly Bulletin of the Ministry of Health and the Public Health Laboratory Service* (June 1948): 136–44.

48. G. Wilson, "Chairman's Summing-Up, Symposium on Food Microbiology and Public Health," *Journal of Applied Bacteriology* 18 (1955): 629.

49. As the Museum began to do with the proceedings of the *Health Matters* conference held a year before opening: G. Lawrence, ed., *Technologies of Modern Medicine* (London, 1994).

Ken Arnold

Museums and the making of medical history

Introduction

Most of the contributions to this volume are based on an implicit faith in
the power of objects to tell, or at least to ask, historians things that the
written word alone cannot.[1] What this range of studies reveals is the vital
and often unique historical evidence that seemingly mute objects can be
made to yield, especially about what people actually did and felt, rather
than just what they wrote or said about their experiences.[2] Taking a step
back from the objects themselves, this essay looks at the places in which
most of them are found – namely medical museums.

At the heart of this essay lies the conviction, not only that artefacts are
significant, but also that their study is greatly enhanced by an understanding
of the history of the museums that keep them; indeed, that researching the
material culture of medicine without an interest in the type of institutions
that preserves it would be to share some of the myopia of ignoring three-
dimensional evidence altogether. It is the nature and history of medical
museums that distinguishes their objects from mere collections of generic
types and odd examples: they provide the essential context that enables lumps
of brute matter – instruments, wax models, pieces of furniture, anatomical
specimens and so forth – to come to life as parts of cultural and social history.

In practice, this insistence on the importance of the history of medical
museums in addition to their contents necessitates research into the
histories of the buildings they occupy, along with the ways in which their
collections were amassed and what has happened to them since they arrived
in the museums. Frequently, of course, buildings housing medical museums
have strong associations with important medical figures or institutions.
In these cases, the additional study that I am advocating comes down, as
J. T. H. Conner has pointed out, to treating medical buildings themselves
as simply particularly large and complicated, but also often well
documented, museum artefacts, capable of revealing much historical insight
in their own right.[3]

What follows cannot hope, and does not seek, to provide an exhaustive
description, or even an inventory, of the huge numbers of institutions
throughout the world that might be classified as medical museums.[4]
Instead, it aims to survey the broad features of the medical museum
landscape, highlighting in particular their role in medical history, and the
legacy of that history in the provision of different types of medical
museums today. The final section of this essay will analyse the types of
medical history presented in these museums, and suggest opportunities for
a more vigorous approach to presenting objects within them.

Museums and the History of Medicine

Early-Modern Experimental Museums

Many of Europe's first museums were, in fact, set up in the apartments and workplaces of medical men. In Italy, then in Northern Europe, and finally in England, Renaissance apothecaries and physicians – along with other emergent professionals and that part of the nobility intent on cloaking itself in the pretensions of "virtuosity" – gathered and studied "natural" and "artificial" curiosities, many of them brought back from travels to unfamiliar countries. Not content simply to hoard and admire their treasures, a number of these early collectors also turned their museums into houses of experience and experimentation. They tasted and tested their specimens, explored the magic of loadstones, assessed the plausibility of theories about fossil origins and, of particular significance here, attempted both to deepen knowledge of *materia medica* and to practise anatomical dissections.[5]

Two legacies of this era of museum history are evident in many of today's medical museums. One is the array of natural historical specimens relating to pre-nineteenth-century medications, particularly the armadillos, alligators, mummified flesh, human skulls and narwhal horns frequently displayed in the "early apothecary shops" common in many local history museums throughout Europe. Possibly the fullest such presentation can be found in Heidelberg's Pharmaceutical Museum. The other legacy lies in the anatomical wax models, or moulages, often represented in older and more comprehensive medical museums. The classic example is the Leiden anatomical collection associated with the anatomical theatre, originally created by Pieter Paaw (1564–1617).[6]

Museums and Medical Education

Medical wax models continued to be made and used for didactic purposes – augmenting the use of cadavers – well into the twentieth century.[7] The eighteenth century, in particular, witnessed elaborate, and some audaciously fanciful, developments in the art of their creation. Over a thousand specimens of anatomical and obstetrical wax models can, for example, be found in the Vienna Institute of the History of Medicine at the Josephium. Other significant collections exist in Florence, in Dresden at the Hygiene Museum, and at the Museum of Morbid Anatomy of Bologna.

The technique of moulaging was particularly useful in rendering accurate models of soft tissue. An especially skilful exponent of the technique of injecting material into tissues to preserve them was the Amsterdam anatomist, Frederik Ruysch (1638–1731), who let his extraordinary imagination loose in juxtaposing specimens so as to create quite breathtaking still-life montages, many of which are still preserved in the Military-Medical Museum of St Petersburg, where Peter the Great deposited them. At least two examples are also still in the Anatomy Museum of Leiden, along with many more prepared by his contemporaries and successors.

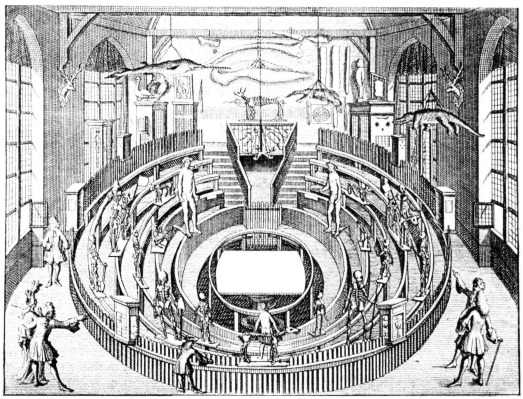

De Anatomie te Leiden.

Figure 1. Leiden Anatomy Theatre. Line Engraving. Even in the seventeenth century, anatomy theatres like this were also used as museum spaces. That in Leiden famously displayed skeletons of Adam and Eve mounted on horse-back.

The most notable exponent of the art in nineteenth-century England was Joseph Towne, whose anatomical and dermatological waxes can be seen in the Gordon Museum in Guy's Medical School.

With notable exceptions, the use of medical museums for research purposes – be it anatomical, natural historical or pharmaceutical – diminished from its height in the sixteenth and seventeenth centuries. The awe-inspiring range of early-modern museum-based experiments and enquiries was reduced to a more or less monolithic concern with taxonomy. At the same time, medical museums became focused on an educational function. In many eighteenth-century medical schools, collections were increasingly seen as essential elements of the curriculum, and a number of important medical museums owe their foundation to this pedagogical purpose.[8]

In England, the Hunter brothers, for example, both exercised passions for collecting and curating. John's collection embodied what he held to be an unwritten book illustrating and summarising a new theoretical approach to the "Animal Oeconomy;" William's museum was more explicitly set up as a resource for anatomical teaching.[9] Parts of both collections survive today at the Hunterian Museum in Glasgow and the Royal College of Surgeons of England in London. Another London medical museum – that

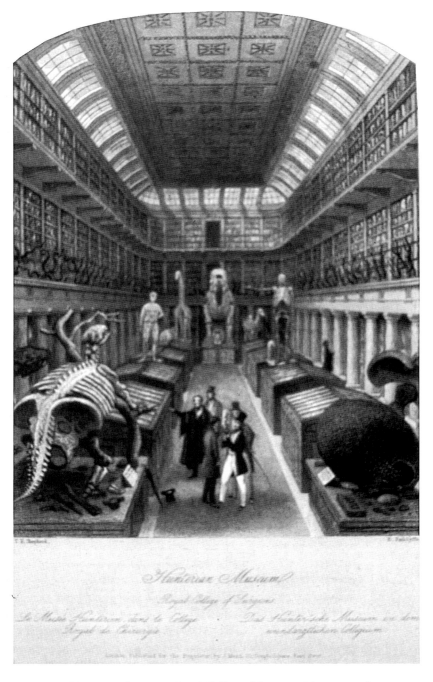

*Figure 2. Hunterian Museum. Royal College of Surgeons. Engraving after
Thomas H. Shepherd, c.1830. The gesticulations of the figures in the foreground
indicate how the collections were used for didactic and demonstration purposes.*

of the Royal Pharmaceutical Society of Great Britain – was also started as a teaching collection, by the Society's School of Pharmacy.

By the end of the nineteenth century, most learned medical societies had gathered some sort of teaching collection; parts of a good number survive today. These include: the Gordon Museum, which is still used by Guy's Medical School in London; the Mütter Museum of the College of Physicians of Philadelphia;[10] and the Warren Anatomical Museum, assembled initially by Dr John Collins Warren between 1850 and 1950 in Harvard Medical School. Warren's most famous exhibit is the "Crowbar Skull," the preserved head of one Phinias Gage, who in 1848 survived massive head injuries from a iron tamping rod that passed through his forehead, and whose mother was encouraged to contribute her son's skull and the tamping bar to the museum in 1866, some five years after his death. This exhibit survived, but many more did not, for the museum has largely been disposed of; even as a teaching forum, this museum had more than its fair share of the marvellous, the wondrous and the ghoulish, and in a modern age of "objective" science, the usefulness and even the propriety of keeping the collection became impossible to defend.[11]

Museums and Public Health Education

The twentieth century has seen a number of developments within medical museums. For much of the first half of the century, they became, in the hands of national states and local governments, widely used as tools for public education in health, sanitation and hygiene. In 1922, for example, Dr Charles Whitebread opened a public health gallery in the Smithsonian Institution in Washington DC. Thirty-five years later, a new *Hall of Health* was opened – its most memorable exhibit being the "transparent woman" or "talking lady," as it was known: a female mannequin with internal organs that lit up while being commented upon by prerecorded descriptions. In Britain, the best known example was Parkes' Museum of Hygiene, founded in 1879, which into the 1950s was still presenting instructional exhibits "in all matters connected with public health."[12] Numerous other examples were established by colonising countries throughout their dominions. They remain popular as educational tools in developing countries.

Museums of the History of Medicine

The other main trend that has, in the twentieth century, led to a virtual explosion in both the numbers and types of medical museum has been a self-conscious concern with the history of medicine. Often associated with, and inspired by, the passions of retired medical men, these museums have grown up alongside, but mostly separate from, the development of an academic interest in the history of medicine. These newer museums have as their aim a determined attempt to understand medicine's past as a significant part of human endeavour. In older medical museums, established collections gradually became historically significant, while, in

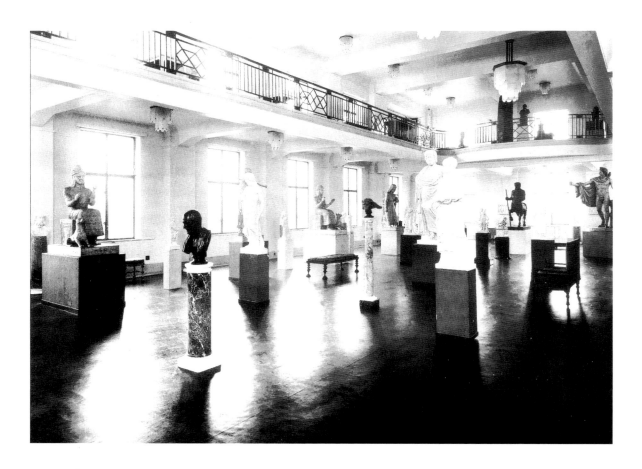

Figure 3. The Hall of Statuary in Henry Wellcome's Historical Medical Museum in the 1930s. Wellcome's passions, not to mention his wealth, allowed him to change the face of medical museums.

more recent examples, collections have been gathered *because* of their historical interest.

Among these recent museums, five types can be identified, each tending to be placed within a characteristic location: those collected and set up by medical entrepreneurs, often found in privately funded institutional venues; those gathered about the biographical locus of individual medical figures established in historic sites; others inaugurated by professional medical bodies and societies located on their premises; yet others emerging from the repositories of particular institutions; and finally, those attached to more broadly based museums.

One man with an extraordinary passion, and almost unlimited funds, single-handedly changed the face of medical museums and collecting in the early part of the century. When Henry Wellcome opened his Historical Medical Museum in 1913, it virtually filled 54A Wigmore Street in London with its halls of "Primitive Medicine" and "Statuary," galleries of "Pictures" and "Ancient Manuscripts, Printed Books, etc.;" front and back ground floors of reconstructed pharmacies, hospitals and the like; not to mention further displays in corridors and on stairs.[13] This was the collection of medicine's material culture on a heretofore unimagined scale – rapidly becoming larger than many of Europe's national cultural collections. Astoundingly, even this was seen by Wellcome as only part of his "Museum of Man."[14] Wellcome died without completing his visionary project, but even the initial task of comprehensively cataloguing the enormous collections he did amass (less more than half that were dispersed after his death) continues as a major project today.

Wellcome's use of a fortune made in the commercial medical world to invest in historical collections was repeated by a number of other entrepreneurs, some in direct imitation, although none on the same scale. The Dittrick Museum in Cleveland, Ohio, was considerably influenced by Howard Dittrick's impressions of Henry Wellcome's museum.[15] The Thackray Medical Museum in Leeds was funded by the proceeds of the sale of a medical supply company, and inspired by the efforts of the grandson of the company's founder, Paul Thackray. In Germany at the beginning of the century, the Hygiene Museum in Dresden was founded by the owner of the Odol-Mouthwash company, Karl August Lingner (*see* Chapter 2, pp. 31–61), and the German Aesculap Works Company, one of the oldest manufacturers of surgical instruments in the world, diverted some of its profits into collecting medical instruments, for the company museum in Tuttlingen.[16]

One popular approach to the writing of medical history has been biographical, and it is not surprising that a good number of medical museums have similarly developed around the life stories of individual medical figures. Down House in Kent, for example, contains the Charles Darwin Memorial Museum. Darwin died in this house and visitors are able to look around the Old Study, where he did much of his work, and to walk along his "thinking path." The Jenner Museum in Gloucestershire is established in the house where Edward Jenner, discoverer of vaccination, died. In it are preserved his personal possessions and material relating to his work, including artefacts from the life of James Phipps, the boy he first vaccinated. In London, one can visit the Florence Nightingale Museum, the Alexander Fleming Laboratory Museum – set up in the laboratory where he did his pioneering work on penicillin, and the house where Sigmund Freud lived after fleeing Vienna.

Away from England, in Budapest, the birthplace of Ignac Semmelweis has been turned into a museum dedicated to the man who discovered that doctors were responsible for passing on puerperal fever to women who had given birth. In Leiden, there is a museum devoted to Boerhaave, the eighteenth-century medical systematist. In France, the celebrated physiologist, Claude Bernard, is the subject of two museums – one in his birthplace, the other in the family mansion of the farm where he was born.[17] The Pest House Medical Museum in Lynchburg, Virginia, is set up in the more modest 1840s white-frame building that was the medical office of a Dr John Jay Terrell during the American Civil War. The Pasteur

Museum in Paris is unusual in both preserving the memory of a great scientist and presenting a type of scientific research that has continued to be practised in his name till today – the latter being the focus of a second structure inaugurated in 1986 in Marnes-la-Coquette (the Museum of Applications of Pasteurian Research).[18]

Professional associations have also supported museums. Typical of this genre of medical museum are the Museum of Pharmaceutical History in Basel, the German Pharmaceutical Museum in Heidelberg, the Göttingen collection of obstetrical and perinatal artefacts, the British Dental Association Museum, and, back in Germany, the Dental History Museum in Cologne.[19]

Some hospitals, such as the Glenside Hospital in Bristol and the Royal London Hospital, have established collections based on their own history. The numbers of such collections may increase significantly in Britain if established plans for re-organisation of the hospital services continue to be implemented. There have been several proposals for converting old hospitals into museums, most notably the suggested use of St Bartholomew's Hospital in London as a museum of national history, which would augment the recently established small museum dedicated to the history of the hospital.

An important part of the history of many of these institutional museums is a period of obscurity, the sense of near loss heightening the precariousness of rediscovery. Two anecdotes exemplify the point. In 1991, a first-year Yale University medical student, Christopher Wahl, found, almost by accident, a collection of about 600 preserved brains and associated photographic material, stored and largely forgotten for nearly 40 years in a former bomb shelter. The material had been gathered by Harvey Cushing, a Yale professor known as "the godfather of neurosurgery," who died in 1939. The collection, now known as the "Cushing Tumor Registry," subsequently went on display. In Southwark in London, the Old Operating Theatre Museum and Herb Garret announces itself as "London's most intriguing historic interior." The roof garret of an eighteenth-century church, containing Britain's oldest preserved operating theatre, was largely forgotten after its premises were taken over by the Post Office and its doorway bricked up early in the twentieth century. Rediscovered in 1956, it has subsequently been restored and converted into a museum.[20]

The Army Medical Museum in the USA provides a very different example of an institutional medical museum. It was founded in 1862 by Surgeon General William Hammond, who directed army medical officers to collect the remains of soldiers on Civil War battlefields and send them back to Washington in order to help the study of military medicine and surgery – what Dr Howard Karsner, writing in 1946, called the pathology of the entire army of a great country. One of its most famous exhibits is the shattered and severed leg of General Daniel Sickles, who, after losing the limb at Gettysburg, attached a note to it and packed it off to the museum

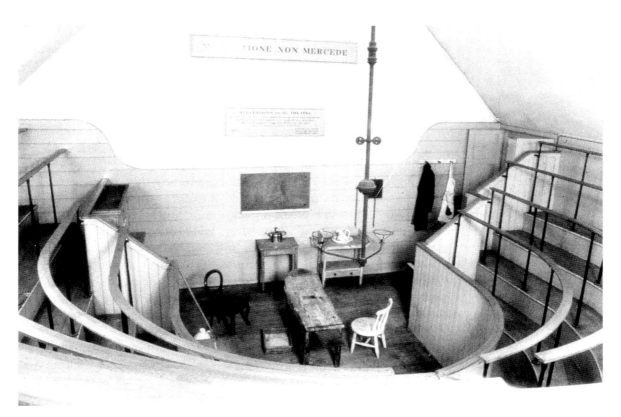

Figure 4. The interior of the Old Operating Theatre, Museum and Herb Garret. A modern museum of the history of medicine that draws its strength from a medical space that lay forgotten and hidden for decades.

in a coffin-like container. Other star attractions of the collection include the bullet that ended Abraham Lincoln's life, and a specimen from the body of his assassin. A year after the assassination, the museum was moved to Ford's Theatre, where Lincoln had been shot. At the end of its first century of collecting, the museum had more than a million specimens, with a further 200 or so more arriving every day.[21]

What is relatively unusual about the Army Medical Museum is its role as an intellectual centre alongside its research activities. By the 1870s, with the Philosophical Society holding its meetings there, the museum had become a focus of intellectual and scientific life in Washington. In the 1880s, the museum's emphasis changed to that of a more general museum of medicine and medical science. The general acceptance of the idea that microbes transmitted diseases resulted in the museum becoming a repository for microscopes and their slides. In the early part of the twentieth century, museum staff were also involved with significant army medical investigations into yellow fever and typhoid; in fact, the first vaccine against typhoid was developed at the museum. During the First World War, the museum was used to produce instructional motion pictures and lantern slides. Thereafter, relations with the medical professions were renewed, particularly with a large-scale project creating a pathology registry.

After the Second World War, the museum became part of the Armed Forces Institute of Pathology. The museum, however, was not a primary part of the Institute's activities, and was destined to be separated from its research concerns. The challenge for the present-day curators of the National Museum of Health and Medicine is to weave a public museum (the USA's largest medical museum) out of the constituent elements cumulatively left over from this extremely rich institutional history.[22]

To complete this overview of the more recently created medical history museums, it is necessary briefly to mention those that comprise a part of those museums having much broader historical or technical perspectives. These include the "reconstructed street" museums – such as the York Castle Museum and Blists Hill Open Air Museum in Ironbridge Gorge. Most are set in the mid to late nineteenth century and feature dispensaries, pharmacies, and doctors' and dental surgeries. Museums that seek to treat the entire history of science often also have collections relating to the medical sciences. The Museum of the History of Science in Oxford, for example, has medical and dental instruments, wet specimens, some wax and ivory models, patent medicines, early X-ray tubes and an early artificial elbow joint.

At the national level, significant collections exist in most science and history museums. The medical collections in the Smithsonian Institution, for example, form one of its oldest divisions, which started as a drugs and plants display exhibited in the 1876 Centennial Exhibition in Philadelphia. The "history of medicine" collections in the Science Museum in London, to take just one more example, are largely based on the "permanent loan" of the non-library material gathered by Henry Wellcome, mentioned above. More recent acquisition of material has continued to keep the collections up to date, enabling the museum recently to open an exhibition that explores how medicine has changed during the twentieth century: *Health Matters* (*see* Chapter 6, pp. 123–43).[23]

***

The cumulative history of some four centuries of medical museums – a history which I have somewhat artificially divided into an early-modern period of museums used for medical research, a later consolidation of their use in medical education, a late-nineteenth- and twentieth-century attempt to use them for public health education, and finally a virtual explosion of self-consciously "historical" medical museums in the past 70 years – has produced an extraordinarily diverse legacy of types of institutions in which medically significant collections are now held. Many of the institutions and collections extant today, particularly the older ones, have themselves evolved through a series of stages, each of which has imprinted a new identity on the objects kept in the collections. An understanding of these successive meanings, where available, can be crucial to the study of this material.

Although extremely sketchy, even the above outline history indicates the ranges of motivations for founding museums. The importance of this history lies in the potential enrichment it gives to the artefacts that the museums contain. For it should prompt students of this material culture to add to their enquiries new questions: when did an object arrive in an institution and how, why was it brought there in the first place, what use has been made of it since?

Historiography in Medical Museums

Along with the traditional practice of keeping collections and catalogue records of their contents, within medical museums considerable thought has, more recently, been given to the way in which their contents are presented to the public. For the remainder of this essay, I want to focus on various strategies by which museums turn their collections into publicly accessible medical history.

In common with many other types of museum, medical history displays have, in the past two to three decades, witnessed a move away from traditional, long timespan, internal histories of the subject to more contextual and interdisciplinary exhibits. In the former, medicine was assumed to be a fairly monolithic intellectual pursuit, with an internal evolution that could be depicted through a mix of objects, illustrations, captions and text panels. In the latter, a different methodology has emerged, in which exhibitions with medical themes are much more broadly interpreted in the context of other subjects and disciplines: most commonly, aspects of cultural and social history, anthropology and archaeology. Two other significant differences also characterise traditional and thematic styles of presentation. First, the former have tended to be set up as "permanent" galleries – with an envisaged lifespan of five to ten years, which, in reality, often ends up double that – whereas interdisciplinary thematic exhibitions have, instead, commonly been "temporary" shows, on view for a maximum period of one year. Second, the broad-sweep (ancient to modern) histories of medicine have most frequently been based on more or less universal collections of medical artefacts – from early scalpels to modern hypodermic syringes – whereas thematic shows often use objects eclectically drawn from a variety of different collections, not infrequently from outside museums altogether.

Creators of both types of exhibition can be prone to using artefacts simply as illustrative material to support predetermined stories, which, by implication at least, are based on other written sources located elsewhere. The exploitation of thematic exhibitions, however, has encouraged considerable amounts of experimentation with alternative approaches to presenting objects; and it is on the basis of the best of this work that the greatest progress has been made with the idea that objects can actually constitute a form of historical and cultural evidence in their own right.

The remainder of this paper will look in more detail at the methodological issues surrounding the curatorial challenge of forming and presenting medical history in museums. I will first describe a range of the "traditional" universal survey exhibitions, then I will look at a small selection of thematic exhibitions that have significantly departed from this model and, finally, I will consider the issue of how medical galleries and exhibitions can make conscious use of artefacts as a form of material evidence – the very "stuff" of the histories they seek to tell.

Traditional Medical History Galleries: The Universal Survey
Almost every major hub of medical activity boasts an exhibition that aims to encompass nothing short of a universal survey of medical history, while many other "medical capitals" contain national versions of that same story. Christoph Mörgeli's description of the Museum of the History of Medicine at Zurich University sums up the intention behind many such displays: "an overview of the history and evolution of medicine" illuminated by "a varied and fully displayed collection containing objects, dating from the earliest times up to the present, … [which] give visual and palpable evidence of the 'knowledge' of medicine."[24] In London, this historiographic goal of a complete history of medicine is fulfilled by the Wellcome galleries in the Science Museum. In Germany, it is located in Ingolstadt, where a selection of material from the permanent collections has been carefully presented in a building that is itself a historic monument, once housing the city's anatomical institute and medical faculty. In Budapest, the medical museum set up in the birthplace of Ignac Semmelweis similarly directs its visitors through the standard chapter headings in a medical history primer: "Prehistoric and Primitive Medicine," "Medicine in the Ancient Orient," "Greek and Roman Medicine," "Islam and Public Health," up to "Rebirth of Medicine in the 16th and 17th centuries," and so on.[25]

The universal surveys of medical history presented in these displays are, however, commonly influenced by national agendas and local variations. Spain's version (the Museum of the History of Medicine, in Catalonia), for example, deals with the development of descriptive anatomy, not through the standard textbook account of the Renaissance "discovery of the human body," but rather by detailing the introduction of anatomical knowledge at the foundation of the Royal College of Surgeons in Cadiz in 1748 and by placing special emphasis on Spanish "topographical" and "anthropological" anatomy. Similarly, at the National Museum of American History in Washington DC, the emphasis within the health sciences displays has very much been on American-made, -produced or -used material.[26] The Vienna Institute of the History of Medicine at the Josephinum has a number of sections displaying the development of Vienna medicine during the past 200 years, with material relating to the ophthalmological pioneer Georg Joseph Beer (1763–1821), the father of phrenology Franz Joseph Gall (1758–1828), and, of course, Sigmund Freud (1856–1939).[27] The medical history museum of Budapest moves from a standard general medical history to an examination of the emergence of the medical school of Pest and of the discovery by the local hero, Semmelweis, of the causes of puerperal fever. Interestingly, in South Africa, there are two medical historical museums: the Cape Medical Museum and the Adler Museum. The former deals exclusively with Western medicine, whereas the latter does contain a small section on traditional medicine: "Apparel and objects used by the witch-doctor in the diagnosis and treatment of disease." As Andy Brown of the Adler Museum has pointed out, however, this balance far from reflects the practices of the people in South Africa, 95% of whose black population would tend to "visit traditional healers before consulting Western doctors."[28]

In Rome, a general Museum of the History of Medicine is housed in the University "la Sapienza." This example is a large-scale affair, covering 800 square metres on three floors, and using some 10,000 objects to reflect the evolution of medical thinking and technology. In common with those of a number of its counterparts, the Sapienza's displays include a number of reproduced objects, made in order to fill perceived gaps in the story being told. The Karl Sudhoff Institute of the History of Medicine and Natural Sciences in Leipzig, to take one other example, has similarly augmented its collection of medical instruments with a set of reproductions of Roman instruments.[29] This tendency to feel the need to augment displays in which original artefacts are missing with more recently reproduced examples points towards one of the defining characteristics of such approaches to medical history galleries: namely, the inclination to view the role of objects in such exhibitions as primarily one of lending material support to the story being told.

These traditional survey exhibitions have tended to be mounted for an audience envisaged both as lacking any prior knowledge of medical history and as having an interest in following that history as a continuum through century after century. Certainly, just to select the example with which I am most familiar, a few studious hours in the Science Museum's Wellcome galleries would provide a solid foundation for anyone with a casual interest in the history of medicine. It also provides a more palpable and vivid sense of what the physical reality of that history was like than any written text could do, no matter how well illustrated. Much of the more recent work in medical history curation, however, has moved away from these monolithic slices of medical history, exploiting instead smaller thematic exhibitions.

Thematic Exhibitions in Medical Museums
Most of the traditional medical history exhibitions just discussed were put together at least a decade ago, and represent something of a culmination of the most recent phase in the history – outlined above – of the founding of medical history museums. Often growing out of a perceived need to

augment such universal survey galleries, a newer type of thematic exhibition has been the subject of experimentation in the past couple of decades. The intellectual foundations for these shows have tended to come from more radical and interdisciplinary areas of academic research. As temporary displays, these exhibitions have often also provided curators with a license to present objects that otherwise would not normally see the light of day in an unusual angle, sometimes quite literally, or in unexpected, even quite jarring juxtapositions. It is often under these circumstances that otherwise mute material can be seen, or rather heard, at its loudest. Most refreshingly of all, special exhibitions frequently allow curators to draw on and present together material otherwise separated by academic disciplines and institutional boundaries.

The most significant element introduced into such cross-disciplinary exhibitions has been art – both historical and contemporary. One of the more important ventures of this type in recent years was the *L'ame au Corps* exhibition mounted at Le Grand Palais in Paris in 1993. Deliberately bringing together material from art and science collections across Europe, this exhibition traced the preoccupation of post-Enlightenment scientists and artists with the connections between the human spirit and its material envelope: the body. At one juncture in the show, for example, tiered steps and sharply focused spot-lights were used dramatically to present a set of model heads used by phrenologists. Set near them were framed works of art by the likes of Daumier, in which the caricaturists' skills similarly used the shapes of their subjects' heads as their subject matter. Without much more than a prosaic caption or two, this skilful juxtaposition tellingly evoked the moment at which particular forms of "science" and of art briefly shared the same perspective of the same subject – that is, the minutely observed and measured contours of the human head – before being wrought apart by the cultural separation of the worlds of aestheticism and empiricism. Throughout the remainder of the exhibition, a further mass of scientific material – anatomical images and waxes, mechanical models reflecting different theories of the body's inner workings, up to modern molecular models – was brought together with paintings, sculptures, prints and drawings by the likes of Chardin, Gericault, Dadd, Dali, Klimt, Munch and Turner, in an intricately and evocatively interwoven fabric that managed, more beautifully and effectively than any essay or monograph could do, to demonstrate the symbiotic and continually evolving relationship between art and science.

Another recent exhibition – *Ars Medica: Art, Medicine and the Human Condition* – this time drawn exclusively from collections in the Philadelphia Museum of Art, explored the complex relationship between medicine and the visual arts through a very different strategy. The presentation here was entirely of works by many of the most familiar names in the history of Western art: Lucas van Leyden, Durer, Rembrandt, Hogarth, Munch, Rauschenberg and so forth. With carefully researched captions that drew

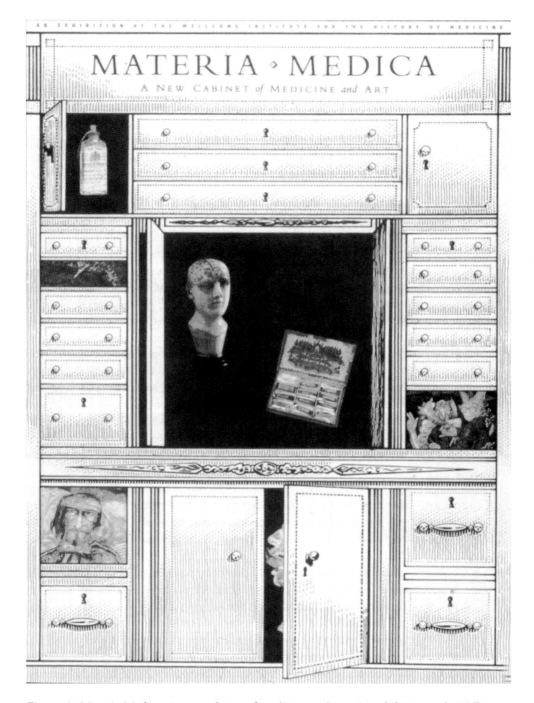

Figure 5. Materia Medica: A new cabinet of medicine and art. *An exhibition at the Wellcome Trust that sought to juxtapose history, art and medicine.*

159   *Ken Arnold   Museums and the Making of Medical History*

out the medical significance of the pieces, the works of art brought to various aspects of medical history the distanced perspective of outsiders to the medical world, but also, more crucially, the careful observation, critical wit, profound wisdom and sheer genius that these artists possessed in such quantity.[30] The point of presenting what might otherwise seem to have been "just an art show" was achieved by the fashion in which the exhibition managed considerably to expand the cultural territory traditionally occupied by medical research and practice and to bring it to the attention of audiences untouched by medical history. The overlaps between the worlds of art and medicine are long-standing and deeply significant for both sides of this now strictly divided pair of disciplines, and this, among other exhibitions, has made it clear that the modern imperative to assign such material to one side or the other has dramatically dulled the full significance of what they truly share.

***

The approach to integrating medical science and art that was adopted in two other recent projects has placed more of an accent on the insights and imaginations of active contemporary artists. *Beyond Ars Medica: Treasures from the Mütter Museum* (1995/96) presented some of the material from this medical history museum and archive alongside photographs by contemporary artists inspired by and developed directly from items in the collection. In the Wellcome Trust's *Materia Medica: A New Cabinet of Medicine and Art* (1995/96), eight working artists were each invited to form a mixed "cabinet" comprising pieces of their own work presented in juxtaposition with material selected from the Wellcome collections (kept in the Wellcome Institute Library and the Science Museum).[31] The rationale behind both these projects was less a matter of exposing areas of medical history to art historical scholarship than an attempt to broaden the approach to material in the history of medicine and, indeed, to expand the range of those usually encouraged to approach it.

A variety of medical museums have, especially during the past five years, opened one or sometimes a series of temporary exhibitions that have done much to explore the history of medicine – exhibitions that have both treated medical science and practice as a cultural activity and examined them in the context of their social relevance to a variety of communities. Constraints of space do not permit even a brief survey of these projects, but one institution in particular exemplifies just how much can be done through a thematic, interdisciplinary approach to aspects of medical history that touch the lives of ordinary people. The German Hygiene Museum in Dresden, with its own fascinating institutional history, has been responsible for some of the most innovative and provocative work in this area, and certainly for the largest output of temporary exhibitions within the area of medical history. A list of just some of its projects can be taken as representative of the many other excellent exhibitions that an essay of this length does not allow me to mention.

The sheer range of exhibitions that the Hygiene Museum has mounted in the past few years hints at the breadth of vision of this pioneering institution. The subjects tackled have included asbestos (*Asbest: zur Geschichte eines Umweltproblems*), rubber (*Gummi: die Elastische Faszination*), drugstore advertising in the GDR (*In aller Munde*), a history of abortion (*Unter anderen Umständen*), the technical and cultural aspects of refrigeration (*Unter Null*), Darwin and his cultural and intellectual legacy (*Darwin und Darwinismus*), baths and bathing (*Das Bad*), "the Pill" (*Die Pille*), the river Elbe (*Die Elbe*), sexual abuse of children, the history of homeopathy, AIDS, and explanations of illness from various cultures and at various times, in a show entitled "Sick. How Come?" (*Krankheit. Warum?*). They all have a direct link to medicine, health and its history, but what additionally holds all this outpouring together is a powerful and involving philouseum by means of a permanent collection. Consciously drawing on its own history, the Hygiene Museum's traditional obligations of promoting public health care – that go back to the early 1900s – are brought up to date with an additional objective of presenting the human body as part of a cultural and ecological environment. The strength and breadth of this programme of exhibitions derive from the less publicly visible activities that go on in the organisation: the preservation of existing collections and their augmentation, the promotion of scholarly research, which often contributes directly to the conceptual work behind the exhibitions, and the provision of a forum for health-orientated communication for educators' unions, self-help organisations and branches of local government.

Cumulatively, these exhibitions have done much to alter the face of medical history within museums, making it clear that medical history is a far broader, more flexible and interlinked subject than was ever imagined before: accessible through other sciences, popular culture, the arts, politics and so on. The new approach to an eclectic range of heretofore unimagined themes has grown up alongside a more adventurous perception of how artefacts might be presented – that is, a revised sense of what the objects actually mean and can tell the public about the history of medicine when they are put on display.[32] This is the subject of the final section of this essay.

Medical Museums and the "Stuff" of History

Medicine touches a special, and especially sensitive, part of our psychological make-up. Consequently, as a medical history curator, one tries in vain entirely and unequivocally to separate the "serious" subject of medicine from the "trivial" response to "blood and guts." We feel medical history through its artefacts, not only, like everything else that has a third dimension, because that history tangibly engages another of our senses, but because many of those objects manage to reach inside us in a most discomforting way – often because they literally relate to our hidden insides. It is this chilly delight that gives special resonance to Ulrich Tröhler's claim that historical medical artefacts – those relating to obstetrics are his particular concern – "may lead us to study *what was felt*."[33]

Many curators of medical collections have been tempted to try to avoid, or even wilfully to prevent, the visceral responses that some visitors might have to medical historical displays. Two-headed babies, shrunken heads and the feet of Egyptian mummies are thus selectively removed to reserve collections. The National Museum of Health and Medicine in Washington DC, for example, has for many years sought to rid its displays of any carnival-show type of attractions, replacing them instead with interactive and didactic exhibitions on the modern medical understanding of our bodies and health. Although there is, of course, a perpetual need to be watchful that a healthy exploration of a difficult subject does not slip into the thoughtless exploitation of strong material, this sensational aspect of medical history surely provides a key to the special significance of the whole subject. An excessively cautious and fearful approach to such displays thus runs the risk of substituting packages of worthy but uninteresting education for windows on to the real world. It also, incidentally, runs the risk of misrepresenting past periods of scientific investigation, which genuinely were energised by a sense of the marvellous and the bizarre.[34]

For this reason, exhibitions with a medical history content, in no matter what museological context – traditional thousand-year-long survey galleries or temporary thematic exhibitions – will, more probably than not, contain objects having a potency that inevitably interrupts and rises above the narrative flow of an exhibition. Two examples taken almost at random from very different types of medical history exhibitions will suffice to make the point. One discovers little extra factual information about the fairly well-known story of President Lincoln's assassination by visiting the Armed Forces Medical Museum in Washington DC, but, as the newspaper critic, Hank Burchard, has described it: "no history text, can make the tragedy as immediate and real as [the fragments of his skull] and the army pathologist's ... heartbroken but graphic official autopsy report" on display there. Similarly, in the Red Cross Museum in Geneva, among a display that is largely made up of exquisitely lit reconstructions, beautiful illuminated text panels, and highly sophisticated slide-shows telling broad brush-stroke stories of health care from pre-history up to the founding of the Red Cross movement, there is something altogether more profound about the impact of a gigantic room filled with the card index of the seven million First World War prisoners of war.[35]

Even though, as just suggested, medical history has privileged access to the core emotions such objects touch, these artefacts are inevitably few and far between. For the most part, both traditional galleries and thematic exhibitions tend to present heavily scripted stories in which objects are mostly used to illustrate, enliven and make palpable a history vouchsafed by textbooks and academic monographs and journals.[36] That said, even with the somewhat diluted faith placed in objects that so many medical history displays embody, the stories they present cannot help but be different from those found in standard textbooks, for they inevitably have greater gravity and more emotional charge, and, especially for those without any background knowledge, they still have the potential to stop visitors in their tracks.

As is admirably indicated by other contributions to this volume, however, more recent work with the material culture of medical history has resulted in much more sophisticated attention being paid to the issue of what objects can, in their own right, uniquely divulge about the history of medicine. Although the use of this approach to artefacts within exhibitions is still in its infancy, any number of object types suggest themselves as material ready to be exploited in more artefact-led exhibitions that could be used to shed extra and unique light on aspects of the history of medicine: surgical and diagnostic instruments to provide insight into the "hands-on" practice of medicine; moulages to act as windows on to particular aspects of medical education; human specimens to open up difficult and sometimes troubling parts of medical history; patient-produced artwork to reveal something of the user's experience of medicine (especially that of the mind); medical posters and public education films to elucidate the understanding of public health policy; army medical collections to suggest both the crucial part played by warring governments in medicine and the nature of injuries and fatalities during war; pharmaceutical products and packaging to explore the commercial context of medicine; instruments of investigation such as microscopes to uncover the methodology of medical research; the attire and costume of medical practitioners to indicate the social and cultural place of various branches of medicine; and collections of medical illustrations to document both the evolution of anatomy, and the relationship between anatomy, physiology, pathology and so forth. This long, but by no means complete, list indicates just how much could be done with such an approach. A brief examination of the first four of these categories might serve to demonstrate how the insights afforded by the study of such material could enrich medical history exhibitions.

Instruments are one of the virtually ubiquitous types of object present in any medical museum. Frequently poorly documented, "the fact that they exist is [as Gretchen Worden has pointed out] often the only available documentation of their existence." Despite the fact that, as Worden goes on to say, "medical historians can exhibit a surprising lack of curiosity when given the opportunity to examine and use an instrument devised by one of the great names in medicine," a significant amount of insight can be teased out of their brute materiality. In the first place, much can be inferred from just how basic the equipment in common use was, and, by implication, the extent of the dexterity of those who successfully made use of it.[37] The mere sight of a seventeenth-century amputation set, with a saw reminiscent of one you might find in a present-day junior carpentry set, conveys a strong sense of the brute physicality involved in such operations at that time. Handling such equipment only helps to drive the point home. Further evidence can be gauged from the development of particular types of equipment – for example, indication of the speed with which new medical ideas and theories were accepted. Thus the increasing use of steel rather than bone handles for surgical equipment offers very direct evidence relating to the notion that diseases were spread by germs that could be excluded by the introduction of sterile environments and equipment.

In addition, as Eduard Caspar Jacob von Siebold, an early curator of the Göttingen collection of perinatal instruments noted as long ago as 1839, "the invented instruments and objects … often speak to us a language more truthful than their inventors by whom they are extolled with all possible hymns of praise." This "language" is in part derived from the emotional impact of a collection such as that displayed in Göttingen: for it is difficult not to empathise with those on whom such instruments were used as much as, if not more than, with those who used them. Medical instruments, in fact, often crystallise the point of contact between practitioner and patient, and consequently have the potential to reveal much about their relationship. One exhibit in the Göttingen collection poignantly illustrates the point: William Smellie's forceps, which he covered in leather so that they might "appear so simple and innocent," or in other words less frightening, to those who endured their effects.[38] Clearly, the sight of a "softer" and more domestic material such as leather covering the bent metal arm used to pull a baby out of its mother's womb was believed to be less distressing than the bare metal, even though the shape and function of the instrument remained unchanged.

Another area of medical history uniquely illuminated by collections of instruments is the context of their manufacture. Even the monotonous ranks of mass-produced instruments, marketed in increasing numbers since the Industrial Revolution, reveal much about the changing organisation of medical practice and education. Not infrequently in earlier periods, medical instruments were either fashioned by innovative practitioners and theoreticians, or custom-made by specially employed instrument makers.[39] The decreasing numbers of such instruments in museum collections is in itself an indication of the change towards a more industrially orientated style of medicine. The numbers of medical instruments found in collections can further indicate the extent of their use; their cost might suggest the range of practitioners that used them; the standard of workmanship in their mechanisms and the accuracy of their calibrations will provide clues to the fashion in which they were expected to be used; and the frequency and fashion in which models were updated may reflect changes in medical ideas and standards of practice.

A second type of artefact found in many medical collections that could potentially provide unique insights into a number of aspects of medical history are moulages, the wax anatomical and dermatological models produced in profusion from the seventeenth century until the mid 1950s. These sometimes quite beautiful sculptures, developed initially for use in anatomy, pathology and obstetrics, were later much utilised by dermatologists. Often made according to the instructions of particular medical tutors or practitioners, by craftsmen with extensive medical knowledge, they can reveal much about the relative development of these various disciplines, and the dominant theories within those fields.

As has been discussed above, a study of moulages can also shed light on the special place that museums have had in the history of medicine. For, unlike so much of the material gathered in today's medical museums, which was inevitably moved from the context in which it was made and first used in order to be added to a museum collection, many wax models are still to be found displayed in the very institutions for which they were created. Thus one can, today, look at the waxes made by Joseph Towne (1806–79) for the Gordon Museum in Guy's Hospital, in that very place. Some examples – such as the pioneering work of Testa Dello Zumbo (1695–1700) in the Muzeo Zoologico de "La Specola" in Florence, the anatomical works by Ercole Lelli in the mid eighteenth century that are to be found in the Anatomical Museum of Bologna University, and the dermatological works in the German Hygiene Museum – are also very significant in what they reveal about the history of the presentation of medicine to a wider, non-professional public. The same significance is to be attached to the didactic plastic mannequins (the transparent men, women and animals) made and exhibited in Europe and America from the 1920s to the 1960s, under whose transparent surface museum visitors could see the internal organs and systems, sometimes lit up, with accompanying audio commentaries (see Chapter 2, pp. 31–61).[40]

A third type of object – which, for publicly accessible museums at least, represents potentially the most difficult exhibits of all – is human specimens. Much museological comment has been passed on the inherent problems of displaying human remains, be they in ethnographic, archaeological or other collections. A rather unusual example highlights the insights that careful investigation of such material in medical collections can reveal. In the anatomical museum of Ferrara University are preserved pieces of human skin bearing tattoos, taken from the bodies of dead prisoners and other convicts who were publicly executed. Claudio Chiarini argues that, far from simply being tokens of the depersonalising, dehumanising process of anatomical investigation, these exhibits can instead be regarded as "graphic voices" capable of transmitting "those desperate invocations, that need for forgiveness, which no one [in their own time] granted." If one agrees with Chiarini, then the display of this particular type of human remain, somewhat counter-intuitively, is to be seen as a partial fulfilment of the "desire for friendship and love that time unfortunately denied" the people from whose bodies they were taken.[41]

Another type of artefact found in a variety of museums, and which potentially represents a source of profound reward for medical historians, are pieces of work, mostly art, produced by patients in medical and mental institutions. Undoubtedly, the most significant body of such material is the Prinzhorn Collection of some 6,000 pictorial objects, held by the Psychiatric Clinic of Heidelberg University. Named after the art historian, psychologist and physician Hans Prinzhorn, who worked on the material in the early 1920s, this collection represents an extraordinarily nuanced body of evidence, both about the lives and thoughts of "mentally deranged" patients of the period, and about their classification, care and treatment.[42]

A recent exhibition of the Prinzhorn Collection at the Hayward Gallery in London gave ample testimony to the fantastic art-historical riches that this material contains. Displayed as a straightforward art exhibition of mounted and framed pictures with two-line captions identifying artist and medium, the beauty and intrinsic – albeit sometimes troubling – interest of the works were given the ideal space and viewing conditions in which to speak for themselves. Somewhat extraordinarily, however, no attempt was made to use the exhibition to explore any questions about the institutional, medical, cultural or social context in which the works had been produced. A great opportunity, therefore, still exists to display the material again, this time to bring out a variety of its other significances. In this case, art-historical interests entirely eclipsed the potential medical historical importance of the material; however, it must be said that many of the insights offered by the four categories of medical material culture just surveyed (surgical instruments, moulages, human remains and patient-produced artwork), and indeed all the other object categories listed above, generally remain largely under-exploited even in medical museums.

As the other essays in this volume make clear, some of this potential insight is now being gathered by researchers working with museum collections and, indeed, some of their insights *are* beginning to be presented in exhibitions; but there is much still to do in making medical artefacts actually carry, rather than merely reflect, medical history within exhibitions. One of the easiest ways of furthering both the research into the material culture of medicine and the active presentation of the resultant insights must be the integration of these two museum-based enterprises. Both can but strengthen the other: for the newer style of thematic exhibitions can clearly be enriched by the types of insight into artefacts produced by this new scholarship, while, at the same time, exhibitions can also both stimulate the need to investigate particular items in a collection and provide the site at which to attempt to put across the results of this research to more than just a clique of other medical historians. Given the thrust of argument in this paper concerning the role of museums in the making and in the preserving of medical history, it is only fitting that such a development should take place in those very same institutions.

Conclusion

Museums must inevitably take the dominant role in preserving and illuminating the historical significance of the material culture of medicine. Along with providing encouragement for in-depth "object" research of the type related in many of the other contributions to this volume, their role, I have argued, has at least two other parts to it. First, their own institutional histories provide crucial contextual information to supplement scholarly pursuit of that nature. Second, by presenting their objects, museums inevitably give them a historiographic role. While most collections of medical objects are still organised according to the conventions of a predetermined history, I have argued that much more is possible by focusing on types of material that have their own story to tell, and in particular by the imaginative use and juxtaposition of this material and the insights it carries within thematic temporary exhibitions. If medical objects are held to have a historical voice, the role of museums is not just to keep them audible but, rather, to make them sing.

Notes

1. For general discussion of this point see, for example, James M. Edmonson, "Learning from the Artefact: Surgical Instruments as Resources in the History of Medicine and Medical Technology," *Caduceus* 9, no. 2 (1993): 87–98; Ghislaine Lawrence, "The Ambiguous Artefact: Surgical Instruments and the Surgical Past," in *Medical Theory, Surgical Practice: Studies in the History of Surgery*, ed. Christopher Lawrence (London, 1992), pp. 295–314; and Gretchen Worden, "Steel Knives and Iron Lungs: Medical Instruments as Medical History," *Caduceus* 9, no. 2 (1993): 111–18. As surgeons and not historians, Angela Faga and Luigi Valdatta have spoken interestingly of the implicit faith in the significance and pleasure of seeing museum objects that is shared by many non-historians. Angela Faga and Luigi Valdatta, "Contribution of the Museum for the History of Pavia University for the Knowledge of Plastic Surgery," in *Proceedings of the Fourth Congress of the European Association of Museums of History of Medical Sciences*, ed. Museo per la Storia dell' Universita di Pavia (Milan, 1988), p. 53.
2. This common enough observation is, for example, made by James Edmonson in his account of the Dittrick Museum of Medical History. James Edmonson, "Dr. Dittrick's Museum," *Caduceus* 6, no. 3 (1990): 1; and by Ulrich Tröhler in his "Tracing Emotions, Concepts and Realities in History: The Göttingen Collection of Perinatal Medicine," in *Non-Verbal Communication in Science Prior to 1900*, ed. Renato G. Mazzolini (Florence, 1993), p. 373.
3. The Old Operating Theatre Museum in Southwark in London provides a particularly strong example of a museum that in effect presents just one large artefact: namely the building itself. As Martin Lipp has shown for the USA, a medical landscape can be traced out on an ordinary map simply by highlighting significant landmarks, and then embellishing it with the theatre of medical history displayed in medical museums. The sites that form such a geographically based history can be as simple and eloquent as the granite gravestone of Mary Mahoney (America's first black trained nurse) in Boston or as deceptively silent as the Ether Monument, again in Boston, which does not name any of the discoverers of anaesthesia because who should be credited was the subject of such bitter controversy. Martin R. Lipp, *Medical Landmarks USA: A Travel Guide* (New York, 1991), pp. 71, 104 and passim.
4. No single volume yet published systematically lists, let alone describes, medical museums throughout the world. The range of institutions in Britain is well covered in Sue Weir, *Weir's Guide to Medical Museums in Britain* (London, 1993), while for the USA Martin R. Lipp (n. 3 above), and though now out of date, the appendix on "Museums of Medical History," in Henry E. Sigerist, *A History of Medicine* (Oxford, 1951), remain useful sources of information on the world's more important medical museums.

5. Paula Findlen, *Possessing Nature: Museums, Collecting, and Scientific Culture in Early Modern Italy* (Berkeley, 1994); Ken Arnold, "Cabinets for the Curious: Practicing Science in Early Modern English Museums" (Ph.D. diss., Princeton University, 1992).

6. W. J. Mulder and H. Beukers, "Injected Specimens in the Anatomy Museum of Leiden," in *Proceedings of the Fifth Colloque of the European Association of Museums of History of Medical Sciences,* ed. Fundacio-Museu d'Histora de la Medicina de Catalunya (Barcelona, 1990), p. 9.

7. Thomas Schnalke, *Diseases in Wax: The History of the Medical Moulages* (Berlin, c. 1995).

8. For accounts of the history of medical museums, see John Pickstone, "Museological Science? The Place of the Analytical, Comparative in Nineteenth-century Science, Technology and Medicine," *History of Science* 32 (1994): 118–21, and Ken Arnold, "Time Heals: Making History in Medical Museums," in *Making Histories in Museums,* ed. Gaynor Kavanagh (London, 1996).

9. See W. D. I. Rolfe, "William and John Hunter: Breaking the Great Chain of Being," in *William Hunter and the Eighteenth Century Medical World,* ed. William Bynum and Roy Porter (Cambridge, 1985).

10. See Gretchen Worden, "The Mütter Museum of the College of Physicians of Philadelphia," in *Beyond Ars Medica: Treasures from the Mütter Museum* (New York, 1995).

11. William Bennett, "Dr Warren's Possessions," *Harvard Magazine* (July/August 1987): 24–31.

12. *Guide to London Museums and Galleries* (London, 1953), p. 10; Audrey B. Davis, "The History of the Health Sciences at the National Museum of American History," *Caduceus* 4, no.1 (1988): 59–71.

13. *Historical Medical Museum Organised by Henry S. Wellcome* (London, 1913).

14. The best account of Henry Wellcome's collecting activities is to be found in Ghislaine Skinner, "Sir Henry Wellcome's Museum for the Science of History," *Medical History* 30 (1986): 383–418. An account of the subsequent history of Wellcome's museum can be found in Georgina Russell, "The Wellcome Historical Medical Museum's Dispersal of Non-Medical Material, 1936–1983," *Museums Journal* 86 (Supplement 1986).

15. James Edmonson (n. 2 above).

16. "Museum der Aesculap-werke AG," in *Proceedings of the Third Congress of the European Association of Museums of History of Medical Sciences,* ed. Deutsches Medizinhistorisches Museum Ingolstadt (Ingolstadt, 1986), p. 249.

17. A. Opinel, "Le Musée Claude Bernard," in *Proceedings of the Fifth Colloque of the European Association of Museums of History of Medical Sciences,* ed. Fundacio-Museu d'Histora de la Medicina de Catalunya (Barcelona, 1990); Jacqueline Sonolet, "Musée-maisons Claude Bernard," in *Proceedings of the Fourth Congress of the European Association of Museums of History of Medical Sciences,* ed. Museo per la Storia dell' Universita di Pavia (Milan, 1988), p. 301.

18. A. Perrot, "Deux musées de l'institut Pasteur, deux conception muséologiques," in *Proceedings of the Fifth Colloque of the European Association of Museums of History of Medical Sciences,* ed. Fundacio-Museu d'Histora de la Medicina de Catalunya (Barcelona, 1990), pp. 189–93.

19. Ulrich Tröhler (n. 2 above); Marielene Putscher, "Museum des Bundesverbandes der Deutschen Zahnarzte," in *Proceedings of the Third Congress of the European Association of Museums of History of Medical Sciences,* ed. Deutsches Medizinhistorisches Museum Ingolstadt (Ingolstadt, 1986), p. 246.

20. Jonathan Welsh, "Many Special Minds are Found at Yale," in *The Wall Street Journal,* February 15, 1996; *The Old Operating Theatre, Museum and Herb Garret: Museum Guide* (London, 1995).

21. For a general introduction to the extraordinary history of the Armed Forces museum, see Robert S. Henry, *The Armed Forces Institute of Pathology, Its First Century* (Washington DC, 1964). A more recent journalistic account has been written by Alan Green, "No Guts, No Glory," *Washington City Paper,* February 1993.

22. Robert S. Henry (n. 21 above). More information can also be found by visiting http://www.sgi.com/Technology/WalterReed_Museum.html.

23. Audrey B. Davis (n. 12 above), pp. 59–71; Brian Bracegirdle, "The Museum of Medical Science in the Year 2000," in *Proceedings of the Fourth Congress of the European Association of Museums of History of Medical Sciences,* ed. Museo per la Storia dell' Universita di Pavia (Milan, 1988), pp. 241–45; Ghislaine Lawrence and Tim Boon, *Health Matters: Modern Medicine and the Search for Better Health* (London, 1994).

24. Christoph Mörgele, *The Museum of the History of Medicine of the University of Zurich* (n.p., 1994), p. 13.

25. Christa Habrich, "Les collections d'étude du musée allemande de l'histoire de la médecine à Ingolstadt," in *Proceedings of the Fourth Congress of the European Association of Museums of History of Medical Sciences*, ed. Museo per la Storia dell' Universita di Pavia (Milan, 1988), pp. 103–07; Jozsef Antall, ed., *Pictures from the Past of the Healing Arts* [*Orvostörténeti Közlemények communicationes de historia artis medicinae*. Supplementum 5], (Budapest, 1972).

26. Filip Cid and Nuria Gorina, "The Museum of History of Medicine of Barcelona, a Conceptual Museum," in *Proceedings of the Fourth Congress of the European Association of Museums of History of Medical Science*s, ed. Museo per la Storia dell' Universita di Pavia (Milan, 1988), pp. 97–102; Audrey B. Davis (n. 12 above), p. 65.

27. *University of Vienna: The Vienna Institute of the History of Medicine at the Josephium*, leaflet edited by Christian Brandstätter (n.p., n.d.).

28. *Alder Museum of the History of Medicine* (Johannesburg, 1980); Andy Brown, "Museum Display – Fractions of a Truth," in *Proceedings of the Sixth Congress of Curators of Museums of the History of Medical Sciences*, ed. Museum Boerhaave Leiden (Leiden, 1992), pp. 149–55.

29. Maria Antonietta Coccanari and Giovanni Benito Scarano, "Le musée d'histoire de la médecine de l'Université de Rome," in *Proceedings of the Fourth Congress of the European Association of Museums of History of Medical Sciences*, ed. Museo per la Storia dell' Universita di Pavia (Milan, 1988), pp. 43–47; Klaus Gilardon, "Medizinhistorische Sammlung des Karl-Sudhoff-Instituts für Geschichte der Medizin und der Naturwissenschaften der Karl-Marx-Universität [Leipzig]," in *Proceedings of the Third Congress of the European Association of Museums of History of Medical Sciences*, ed. Deutsches Medizinhistorisches Museum Ingolstadt (Ingolstadt, 1986), p. 246.

30. Diane R. Karp et al., *Ars Medica: Art, Medicine and the Human Condition. Prints, Drawings, and Photographs from the Collection of the Philadelphia Museum of Art* (Philadelphia Museum of Art, 1985).

31. *Beyond Ars Medica: Treasures from the Mütter Museum*, exhibition catalogue (New York, 1995); Ken Arnold and Martin Kemp, *Materia Medica: A New Cabinet of Medicine and Art* (London, 1995).

32. There is not space here to speculate on how closely linked are the developments of new thematic approaches in exhibitions and new museological attitudes to the presentation of objects. My own suspicion is that the two went virtually hand in hand: the former gave legitimacy to the use of all sorts of objects not before shown in medical history exhibitions, it exposed curators to a variety of disciplines with very different – often far more sophisticated – approaches to material culture, and it encouraged them to experiment in shows that would only last a maximum of a year.

33. Ulrich Tröhler (n. 2 above), p. 373.

34. William Bennett (n. 11 above), p. 31, has described the demise of "a taste for the marvellous" within science museums in his account of the Warren Anatomical Museum in Harvard, Mass.

35. Hank Burchard, "It's Strange Inside the Medical Museum," *The Washington Post,* February 2, 1979, p. 6; *Musée international de la Croix-Rouge et du Croissant-Rouge* (Geneva, 1990).

36. The emblematic museum for the illustrative approach may well be the Institute of History of Medicine in Hyderabad, India. For here, large amounts of the material culture to support the story of medical history are not available in replica, so that the history is instead woven around recent artists' renditions of medical subjects in Indian history. Sample exhibits include "Pictures from Ayurvedic Books" and a "Show-case Showing Replicas of Medical Sciences in the Buddhistic Art." Somewhat refreshingly, the attitude here has not been to worry about the support of material evidence at all, but simply to take a very literal approach to the didactic task of illustrating the history of Indian medicine. D. V. Subbba Reddy, ed., *Institute of History of Medicine: Hyderabad. Museum Guide* [*Indian medicine*] (Secunderabad, c. 1971).

37. Gretchen Worden (n. 1 above), pp. 111–15.

38. Ulrich Tröhler (n. 2 above), pp. 369, 346.

39. An unusual case such as that of the highly specialised instruments made by J. Th. Hoefftcke in the early nineteenth century, kept by the University Hospital in Leiden, may also suggest much about the relative power of instrument makers, users (i.e. surgeons) and medical

theoreticians. Willem J. Mulder, "J. Th. Hoefftcke, University Instrument Maker in Leiden," in *Proceedings of the Third Congress of the European Association of Museums of History of Medical Sciences,* ed. Deutsches Medizinhistorisches Museum Ingolstadt (Ingolstadt, 1986), pp. 125–27.

40. For a history of medical moulages, and the museums that contain them, see Thomas Schnalke (n. 7 above).

41. Claudio Chiarini, "Les 'voix graphiques' du musée anatomique de Ferrare," in *Proceedings of the Fourth Congress of the European Association of Museums of History of Medical Sciences,* ed. Museo per la Storia dell' Universita di Pavia (Milan, 1988), p. 51.

42. *Beyond Reason. Art and Psychosis: Works from the Prinzhorn Collection* [Hayward Gallery exhibition catalogue] (London, 1996). Another very significant collection of such material is held at the Bethlem Royal Hospital, where the names of some of the individual artists are far better known: Richard Dadd, Jonathan Martin and Charles Sims amongst them. The Wellcome Institute Library also contains much material of a similar nature.

Addresses of main museums cited

Austria

Museum of the Institute of the History of Medicine
Museum des Instituts für Geschichte der Medizin
Josephinum
Währinger Str. 25
A-1090 Vienna IX

France

Pasteur Institute
Musée Pasteur
25, rue du Docteur-Roux
Paris Cedex 15
F-75724

Germany

Aesculap Works Museum
Aesculap-Werke AG
Aesculap Platz
D-78532 Tuttlingen

Dental History Museum
Museum des Bundesverbandes der Deutschen
Zahnärzte
Universitätsstr. 71
D-50931 Köln 41

German History of Medicine Museum
Deutsches Medizin–Historisches Museum
Anatomiestr 18/20
Ingolstadt D-85049

German Hygiene Museum
Deutsches Hygiene-Museum
Lingnerplatz 1
D-01069 Dresden

German Pharmaceutical Museum
Deutsches Apotheken-Museum
Bureau, Heidelberg Schloss

Friedrichstr. 3
D-69117 Heidelberg

*Karl Sudhoff Institute of the History of
Medicine and Natural Sciences*
Karl-Sudhoff-Institut für Geschichte der
Medizin und der Naturwissenschaften des
Bereiches Medizin
Universität Leipzig
Augustusplatz 10/11
D-04109 Leipzig

*Obstretrics collection of the University's
women's clinic*
Die Geburtshilflische Sammlung der
Universitäts-Frauenklinik
Ethik und Geschichte der Medizin
Humboldtallee 36
D-37073 Göttingen

Prinzhorn Collection
Prinzhorn Sammlung der Psychiatrischen
Universitäts-Klinik Heidelberg
Voßstr. 4
D-6911 Heidelberg

*Psychiatric Clinic of the
University of Heidelberg*
Postfach 105760
D-69047 Heidelberg

Hungary

*Semmelweis Museum, Archives for the
History of Medicine*
Semmelweis Orvostörténeti
Múzeum, Könyvtar es Levéltar
Apród u 1-3
H-1013 Budapest

India
Institute of History of Medicine in Hyderabad
State Health Museum
11-6-15
Hyderabad 500004

Italy
Anatomical Museum "G. Tumiati"
Museo Anatomico "G. Tumiati"
Dip. Morfologia ed Embriologia
Sezione Anatomia Umana
Via Fossato di Mortara 66
I-44100 Ferrara

Museum of the History of Medicine, "la Sapienza"
Università di Roma "La Sapienza"
Museo di Storia della Medicina
Facoltà di Medicina e Chirurgia
Viale dell'Università 34A
I-00185 Rome

Museum of the History of the University of Pavia
Museo per la Storia dell'Università di Pavia
Strada Nuova 65
I-27100 Pavia

Museum of Morbid Anatomy of Bologna
Museo di Anatomia e Istologia Patologica
Via Massarenti 9
I-40138 Bologna

Muzeo Zoologico de "La Specola"
Museo 'La Specola'
Via Romana 17
I-50125 Firenze

Netherlands
Leiden Anatomical Collection
Anatomisch Museum
Wassenaarseweg 62
NL-2333 AL Leiden (Zuid-Holland)

Museum Boerhaave
National Museum of the History of Science and Medicine
Lange St Agnietenstr 10
NL-2312 WC Leiden

Russia
Military Medical Museum
Voenno-medicinskij Muzej
Lazarentnyj per 2
St Petersburg

South Africa
Adler Museum of the History of Medicine
University of the Witwatersrand
POB 1038
Johannesburg 2000

Cape Medical Museum
POB 16511
Vlaeberg 8018
Cape Town

Spain
The Museum of the History of Medicine of Catalonia
Fundacio-Museu d'Historia de la Medicina de Catalunya
Passatge Mercader 11
ES-08008 Barcelona

Switzerland
Museum of Pharmaceutical History
Schweizerisches Pharmazie-Historisches Museum
Totengässlein 3
CH-4051 Basel

Museum of the History of Medicine of the University of Zurich
Med-historisches Institut
SOC E 14
Rämistrasse 69
CH-8001 Zürich

Red Cross Museum
17 avenue de la Paix
CH-1202 Geneva

United Kingdom
Alexander Fleming Laboratory Museum
St Mary's Hospital
Praed Street
Paddington
London W21NY

Bethlem Royal Hospital Archives and Museum
The Bethlem Royal Hospital
Monks Orchard Road
Beckenham
Kent BR3 3BX

Blists Hill Open Air Museum
Ironbridge Gorge Museum
Telford
Shropshire TF8 7AW

British Dental Association Museum
64 Wimpole Street
London W1M 8AL

Charles Darwin Memorial Museum
Down House
Luxted Road
Downe
Kent BR6 7JT

Florence Nightingale Museum
Florence Nightingale Museum
2 Lambeth Palace Road
London SE1 7EW

Freud Museum
20 Maresfield Gardens
London NW3 5SX

Glenside Hospital Museum
Glenside Hospital
Blackbery Hill
Stapleton

Bristol
Avon BS16 1DD

Gordon Museum in Guy's Medical School
United Medical and Dental Schools (UMDS)
The Wills Library
Guy's Hospital
London SE1 9RT

Hunterian Museum (Glasgow)
University Avenue
University of Glasgow
Glasgow
Strathclyde G12 8QQ

Hunterian Museum (London)
Royal College of Surgeons of England
35–43 Lincoln's Inn Fields
London WC2A 3PN

Jenner Museum
The Chantry
Church Lane
Berkeley
Gloucestershire GL13 9BH

Museum of the History of Science
Broad Street
Oxford OX1 3AZ

The Old Operating Theatre
Museum & Herb Garret
St Thomas's Church
9A St Thomas's Street
London SE1 9RT

Royal College of Surgeons of England
35–43 Lincoln's Inn Fields
London WC2A 3PN

Royal Pharmaceutical Society of Great Britain
1 Lambeth High Street
London SE1 7JN

St Bartholomew's Hospital Archives
St Bartholomew's Hospital
West Smithfield
London EC1A 7BE

Thackray Medical Museum
131 Beckett Street
Leeds
West Yorkshire LS9M 7LP

The Science Museum
National Museum of Science & Industry
Exhibition Road
London SW7 2DD

Wellcome Institute for the History of Medicine
183 Euston Road
London NW1 2BE

York Castle Museum
York YO1 1RY

USA
Dittrick Museum of Medical History
11000 Euclid Avenue
Cleveland
OH 44106-1714

Mütter Museum
The College of Physicians of Philadelphia
19 South 22nd St.

Philadelphia
PA 19103

National Museum of American History
Smithsonian Institution
Washington DC 20560

National Museum of Health and Medicine
Armed Forces Institute of Pathology
Dahlia and 14th Streets NW
Washington DC 20306

Philadelphia Museum of Art
26th St and Benjamin Franklin Pkwy
Philadelphia
PA 19130

The Pest House Medical Museum
Old City Cemetry
711 Old Trents Ferry Rd
Lynchburg
VA 24503

Warren Anatomical Museum
Harvard Medical School Building
25 Shattuck St
Boston
MA 02115

Index